Forever
Young

Forever Young

THE SCIENCE OF
NUTRIGENOMICS FOR
GLOWING, WRINKLE-FREE
SKIN AND RADIANT HEALTH
AT EVERY AGE

Nicholas Perricone, M.D.

ATRIA BOOKS

new york   london   toronto   sydney

ATRIA BOOKS
A Division of Simon & Schuster, Inc.
1230 Avenue of the Americas
New York, NY 10020

First Atria Books hardcover edition September 2010

ATRIA BOOKS and colophon are trademarks of
Simon & Schuster, Inc.

For information about special discounts for bulk purchases,
please contact Simon & Schuster Special Sales at
1-866-506-1949 or business@simonandschuster.com.

The Simon & Schuster Speakers Bureau can bring authors
to your live event. For more information or to book an event,
contact the Simon & Schuster Speakers Bureau at
1-866-248-3049 or visit our website at www.simonspeakers.com.

Designed by Suet Yee Chong

Illustrations by Troy Doolittle

Manufactured in the United States of America

10   9   8   7   6   5   4   3   2

Library of Congress Cataloging-in-Publication Data is available.

ISBN 978-1-4391-7734-1
ISBN 978-1-4391-7737-2 (ebook)

To Nikola Tesla,
scientist, humanitarian, forgotten genius

Contents

Introduction

It seems impossible that my first book, *The Wrinkle Cure,* was published well over ten years ago, but time has a way of doing that. In fact, time seems to go by faster with each passing year. Since the excitement generated by that first book, I have continued to devote myself to slowing down time, or at least the toll it takes on our bodies. In *The Wrinkle Cure,* I introduced the concept that inflammation is at the basis of aging and age-related disease. This inflammation exists over a broad spectrum that ranges from low to high. On the low side, it occurs on a cellular level and is invisible to the naked eye. It can be discerned only microscopically or submicroscopically on a molecular level. On the high end of the spectrum, the inflammation is visibly evident as redness and swelling, as seen in a wound or sunburn.

In *The Wrinkle Cure,* I explained that this low-grade, subclinical, cellular inflammation is ultimately responsible for cell dysfunction, leading to organ dysfunction, aging, and death. In addition, I identified this subclinical inflammation as being the basis of such diverse age-related diseases as atherosclerosis, diabetes, various forms of cancer, Alzheimer's disease, and other neurologic diseases, as well as wrinkling of the skin.

My colleagues and mainstream medicine in general vigorously resisted the concept of the inflammation/aging/disease connection. Fortunately, a great deal has changed in a decade, and in that time, numerous studies have validated this concept. Many therapeutic interventions are now being developed counteracting subclinical inflammation, thereby prolonging both our health and our life span.

The Diabetes/Aging Connection

One of the models I use as an accelerated aging prototype is the disease of diabetes. Studying diabetes has helped me to understand the effects of irregularities in blood sugar and their role in the production of free radicals, leading to glycation and inflammation. Glycation is an inflammatory biochemical process that occurs when a glucose (sugar) molecule binds to a protein molecule without the influence of enzymes. In scientific terms we refer to these sugar/protein bonds as AGEs, an appropriate acronym for advanced glycation end products. Glycation and AGEs are highly damaging to all organ systems, including the skin. AGEs can cause arterial stiffening, atherosclerosis, cataracts, neurological impairment, diabetic complications, wrinkled, sagging skin, and more. **The inflammation and glycation that I observed in diabetics whose disease was poorly controlled resulted in those patients' aging one-third faster than the normal population.**

The Forever Young Approach to Aging

Uncontrolled or poorly controlled diabetes is not the only model for accelerated aging. As we enter a new decade, I am looking at another accelerated aging model. This model has provided me with the information I need to develop novel therapeutic interventions to further slow the aging process and radically decrease the onset of age-related disease. The culprit is an acute, severe, systemic infection known as sepsis, which leads to septic shock, the onset and progression of which closely parallel the bodily changes seen during aging. **Sepsis leads to disorders that take place on a cellular level and closely mimics, in an abbreviated period of time, what happens to our bodies over a period of years and decades in the normal aging process.**

Understanding how we age on a cellular level gives us the information we need to retard or even reverse the process. In *Forever Young* you will learn about the science of nutrigenomics and how some very special foods and substances can alter the way you age, both mentally and physically. **Nutrigenomics is the study of how nutrition affects gene expression and how certain nutrients can turn on the genes that block disease and turn off the genes that cause accelerated aging and disease.** As I have often told my patients, readers, and viewers, the fountain of youth may be no further away than your next meal!

As I observed accelerated models of aging, like poorly controlled diabetes and sepsis, and studied and implemented nutrigenomics, I have developed strategies designed to keep you, if not Forever Young, at least looking and feeling your very best for many decades into the future.

Thank you for joining me on this life-changing journey.

Nicholas Perricone, M.D., F.A.C.N., C.N.S.
Madison, Connecticut
January 2010

Forever
Young

Chapter One

THE ICU:

A NEW ANTIAGING RESEARCH LABORATORY

The day had dawned cold and gray with a lowering sky on the morning of February 16. The dark, angry waves of the Long Island Sound dashed against the rocks, a harbinger of worse to come. Another snowstorm was scheduled for New York and Connecticut, making the winter of 2010 one for the record books from Florida to Maine. Escaping to the tropics was on my mind, but duty called.

This was the day I was turning in the manuscript for my new book, *Forever Young.* I was proud to have written a book that broke new ground yet apprehensive, because the science might be considered cumbersome. I knew that there was no other way to tell the story. People needed strategies to stop the deadly degenerating signs of aging, and I feel it is important to explain my recommendations, which are all scientifically based.

As I nursed a cup of green tea and read the news on the Internet, a 24-point-type headline from the United Kingdom's *Financial Times* caught my eye: "Scientists discover the secret of ageing." The article explained how one of the biggest puzzles in biology—how and why living cells age—had been solved by an international team based at the United Kingdom's Newcastle University. Using a complex "systems biology" approach, the researchers, in conjunction with scientists from the University of Ulm in Germany, had set out to discover why cells become senescent, or, in other words, grow old. The research, published by the journal *Molecular Systems Biology,* showed that when an aging cell detects serious DNA damage, which may be the result of general wear and tear from daily living, it sends out internal signals. These distress signals trigger the cell's mitochondria, the energy-producing part of the cell, to make free-radical molecules, which instruct the cell either to destroy itself or to stop dividing. The reason for this is to avoid the damaged DNA that results in cancer.

As you will discover in these pages, I am convinced that the damaging diseases and cellular destruction associated with aging begin with the mitochondria. I concur with the research findings from Newcastle University, as they validate my own research regarding how and why we age. The release of this study just as I was delivering my manuscript to my publisher was very exciting, because the researchers' discovery echoes the underlying theme of this book.

I have gone beyond the science of why we age to search for practical ways to intervene in the process. In *Forever Young* you will learn new, effective, and safe strategies to protect the mitochondria, the mitochondrial DNA, and other parts of the cell from this programmed cell death, known as apoptosis, starting with the miraculous therapeutic powers of niacinamide (vitamin B3), which you will read about on page 107.

A New Model for Understanding Aging

My first experience with seriously ill patients occurred when I was a medical student at Michigan State University College of Medicine. During my rotation in internal medicine, particularly the weeks spent in the intensive care unit, I became intimately familiar with sepsis, one of the most common causes of death.

Also known as gram-negative bacteremia and gram-positive bacteremia, sepsis occurs when infectious agents like bacteria or fungi or products of infection like bacterial toxins enter the body, most often through a wound or incision. If this systemic infection goes unchecked, it leads to a condition known as septic shock, resulting in hypotension, or extremely low blood pressure; dysregulation of blood sugar; and the failure of such multiple organ systems as the heart, kidney, liver, and lungs.

The Sepsis/Inflammation/Aging Connection

In 1981 when I was in medical school, I was trying to understand what caused underlying damage to the vital organs during septic shock. The question was a huge challenge for both physicians and scientists. The research indicated that metabolic changes occurring on a cellular level were the primary cause of organ dysfunction and failure. The consensus was that these fundamental metabolic disturbances were the result of inadequate tissue oxygenation and a disruption of the body's ability to control blood sugar levels. This combination of symptoms came to be known as multiple organ dysfunction syndrome, or MODS. It was widely hypothesized that multiple organ dysfunction syndrome resulted from tissue hypoxia, a condition in which vital organs do not get enough oxygen to meet their needs. Fast-forward to a new millennium: the concept of inadequate oxygen levels to vital organs as the fundamental cause of MODS *is* now being seriously questioned.

Today, scientists believe that adequate oxygen is delivered to the vital organs by the bloodstream during sepsis and septic shock. The problem is that the cells are unable to use that oxygen, even though it is being supplied at adequate levels. The inability of the vital organs to utilize oxygen is a cellular malfunction in the tiny organelles known as the mitochondria. This impaired cellular oxygen problem is termed *cytopathic hypoxia*. Just as cytopathic hypoxia is far more important in the generation of MODS than had ever been thought in the past, I propose that cytopathic hypoxia, as seen in the cellular changes of aging, is far more important to the degeneration of the organ systems than was previously believed.

Having come to that conclusion, I had to ask the next question: If cells cannot utilize the oxygen, where in the cell is the defect? The answer is the mitochondria.

The Mighty Mitochondria

The mitochondria are tiny energy-generating parts of the cell. They function as microscopic furnaces, converting food into fuel, and are responsible for all energy production in the body. The majority of the oxygen supplied to the cell is utilized by the mitochondria to make a chemical known as adenosine triphosphate, or ATP. ATP is the energy storage and transfer molecule that is essential to life. As I discussed in one of my previous books, *Dr. Perricone's 7 Secrets to Beauty, Health, and Longevity*, functioning mitochondria are vital to maintaining a healthy body and beautiful skin.

A Closer Look at Mitochondrial Function

Although tiny, the mitochondria play a huge role in the body as the energy-producing portion of the cell. To accomplish this feat, they

FREE-RADICAL CHEMISTRY

Many people are confused about free radicals. They know that they are bad and that antioxidants combat them. Understanding the chemistry of free radicals will give you an important perspective on aging.

Atoms and molecules are most stable when there is a pair of electrons circulating in their outer orbit. When a molecule or atom loses one of the electrons, it becomes a *free radical*. Its mission in life has now become the quest for another atom or molecule to hook up with. Any substance that rips electrons away from another molecule is known as an oxidizing agent or electrophile. Free radicals can damage tissues, cell membranes, and DNA, disrupting our store of genetic information, which may lead to the initiation of certain cancers.

Free radicals can also oxidize the fats that make up the cell wall membrane and the membrane covering the mitochondria and the nucleus. This oxidation can lead to cellular dysfunction and serious damage to the immune system and major organs such as the brain, heart, kidneys, and pancreas. Free radicals contribute to at least fifty major diseases, including atherosclerosis, heart disease, rheumatoid arthritis, and lung disease, as well as accelerated aging. Although free radicals exist for only a fraction of a second, the inflammatory cascade that they generate goes on for hours or days.

Antioxidants, including vitamin C, alpha-lipoic acid, and Co Q10, are known as reducing agents. They neutralize free radicals and leave a much more benign antioxidant free radical in its place. Unfortunately, the mitochondria are a site of constant free-radical production (see page 6) and very susceptible to the damage that free radicals can cause. If we hope to preserve youthful function and prevent disease, it is critical to search for agents and antioxidants that will protect the mitochondria from free-radical damage.

consume 90 percent of the oxygen that is needed by our bodies. As mentioned, this oxygen is used to oxidize fuel or burn food to synthesize ATP, which is the energy currency of the cell. This process of ATP production in the mitochondria is known as *oxidative phosphorylation* and takes place in the part of the mitochondria known as the *electron transport chain*. Within the electron transport chain, ATP is produced in five steps. If anything disrupts this chain, free radicals are created; this further disrupts the electron transport chain, causing irreparable damage to the mitochondria. Damage to the mitochondria and disruption of the electron transport chain are the first events seen in sepsis. Unchecked, this results in total systemic collapse, multiple organ failure, and death.

Although it may seem counterproductive, the energy produced by the mitochondria is the major source of free-radical production in the cells. This is a result of the metabolic process that converts food and oxygen to water and ATP. As energy production takes place in the electron transport chain, within the mitochondrial membrane, about 5 percent of the electrons escape. This creates free radicals that damage both the mitochondria and the cell.

Therapeutic Strategies for the Mitochondria in Disease and Aging

Although the concept that free radicals are responsible for triggering an inflammatory response on a cellular and molecular level was considered with skepticism when I introduced it in *The Wrinkle Cure*, it is now dogma accepted by even the most conservative scientists. The idea that free radicals and inflammation cause cellular dysfunction and accelerate the aging process is now considered common knowledge as well.

Strategies for Mitochondrial Protection

If you want to slow down the aging process and keep your body functional at optimal health, you need to protect the mitochondria and your cells from free radicals. Mitochondrial antioxidants and free radical scavengers can counter the damaging effects of an inflammatory cascade.

Mitochondrial Antioxidants and Free-Radical Scavengers

Mitochondrial antioxidants are one therapeutic approach in treating acute sepsis as well as aging. This is of critical importance because *any* damage to the mitochondria results in the loss of energy production. A young cell is characterized by high energy production. Conversely, aged cells are characterized by low energy production and an inability to repair themselves.

Glutathione: The Master Antioxidant

Cells have evolved a defense system to protect against this damage by free radicals. It consists of antioxidants and enzymes that can neutralize oxygen-based free radicals. One of the key substances in cellular protection is glutathione. Glutathione is a tripeptide, a molecule composed of three amino acids, and is the most abundant and important antioxidant protective system in our cells. Critical in the cell's defense against inflammation-generating free radicals and oxidative stress, glutathione comes to the rescue whenever a cell is under severe oxidative stress, as an excess of free radicals is called. The mitochondria depend upon cellular glutathione for protection. Produced in the cytosol, the watery portion of the cell, this glutathione must be transferred into the mitochondria to defend against the free radicals, also known as *reactive oxygen species,*

GLUTATHIONE BREAKTHROUGH

A major breakthrough in the use of glutathione is a recently synthesized molecule that is proving to be extremely protective on a cellular level. This derivative of glutathione is known as *S*-acyl-glutathione. This new molecule is a combination of a fatty acid attached to the glutathione molecule. The combination of a fatty acid with the glutathione enables the glutathione to be easily transported into the cell and subsequently into the mitochondria. This process is similar to the results I have seen using the standard glutathione molecule in my phospholipid carrier system.

One of the new *S*-acyl-glutathione derivatives I have been working with is *S*-palmitoleic glutathione (glutathione combined with palm oil). In several studies, this molecule has been able to enter cells, where it neutralizes such free radicals as reactive oxygen species (ROS). The acyl derivatives of glutathione also provide protection to the cell plasma membrane, the outer fatty portion of the cell. Studies show that they are extremely protective to fibroblast cells, which are responsible for producing collagen and elastin in our skin. Protecting this important part of the cell can lead to more youthful-looking, healthier skin.

In other studies, the *S*-acyl-glutathione derivatives are proving to be protective to brain cells. You will see many examples of substances that are therapeutic to both skin and brain throughout this book. I refer to this phenomenon as the Brain/Beauty Connection.

The Brain/Beauty Connection

During medical school, I spent a good deal of time working with patients who were receiving pharmacological agents for the central nervous system. Each time these patients were given treatment, I observed a markedly improved appearance of their skin. This is understandable if you know the basics of embryology, the branch of biology that studies the growth of the fertilized egg to approximately four months of gestation. During this period, all of the body's organ systems are derived from three distinct and separate layers of tissue in the embryo. **Both the skin and the brain are derived from the same embryonic tissue, which is known as the ectoderm. There is an important and powerful connection between the brain and the skin. It should not be surprising that therapeutic agents that affect the brain positively would also be beneficial to the skin.**

One of the new *S*-acyl-glutathione derivatives I have been working with is *S*-palmitoleoylglutathione (glutathione combined with a monounsaturated fatty acid found in palm oil known as palmitoleic acid), which is an important discovery in the treatment of neurological problems associated with aging such as Alzheimer's disease. Thanks to the brain/beauty connection, they are also extremely efficacious in treating the skin.

Increasing Glutathione Production

Another strategy for providing glutathione to the cell and giving additional protection to the mitochondria is to provide precursors that are needed for the formation of glutathione. One very important precursor is a slightly modified amino acid known as *N*-acetylcysteine (NAC). *N*-acetylcysteine is a derivative of the amino acid ʟ-cysteine. NAC contains a sulfur group known as a thiol, and it is the thiol that gives this amino acid its antioxidant effects. The cysteine portion of NAC is one of the three peptides that make up the glutathione molecule, and because it provides this building block, more glutathione is produced.

In combination with two other amino acids, glutamine and glycine, *N*-acetylcysteine promotes the synthesis of glutathione in the liver. Both *N*-acetylcysteine and alpha-lipoic acid, when administered together (see page 13), are precursors or building blocks of glutathione and work synergistically to elevate glutathione levels in the cell.

Physicians have been administering NAC to patients suffering from acute sepsis to elevate levels of glutathione in the mitochondria and protect against organ failure. Oral supplementation is also an excellent strategy to protect the body as we age.

While I was interning in pediatrics at the Yale University Medical Center, I encountered a problem on more than one occasion in the ER involving children suffering from an acetaminophen (Tylenol) overdose. Acetaminophen is extremely toxic when taken in large doses because it causes liver failure. At the time, the Yale Pediatric ER therapeutic protocol was to have the patient drink a foul-smelling liquid called Mucomyst. Designed to be used in a nebulizer, Mucomyst was a therapy for patients with respiratory problems. It worked by breaking down thick mucus in the bronchials of patients with lung problems. Mucomyst is a solution of *N*-acetylcysteine. The thiol in it is responsible for its terrible rotten egg aroma, because it is a sulfur group. In the Tylenol overdoses, NAC works by elevating levels of glutathione in the liver cells, preventing free-radical damage and liver damage. Although we all pitied the poor children who were forced to drink this horrible-smelling solution, we surmised that after experiencing this drink, they would not go near a Tylenol tablet, unsupervised, for the rest of their lives.

---

or ROSs. It is difficult to overstate the importance of glutathione as the body's primary antioxidant defense system.

Scientists and physicians, myself included, have spent many years researching methods to increase glutathione within the mitochondria. **Elevating glutathione levels and other substances that protect against free-radical damage in the mitochondria is the cornerstone of our quest to look and feel Forever Young.**

One of the greatest challenges in working with glutathione is the fact that glutathione supplementation has not been viable. This is because oral ingestion of supplemental glutathione is rapidly digested by the gastrointestinal system. Fortunately, we are finding ways to circumvent this problem. One such method is the focal point of my own research: the development of a phospholipid carrier system that is capable of transferring glutathione into the cells. This transdermal delivery system allows the mitochondria to receive increased levels of this protective tripeptide. When applied to the skin, glutathione, via the phospholipid carrier, is able to penetrate various levels, reaching into the deep dermis and finally into the subdermal microvasculature, or the small blood vessels under the skin. From this point, glutathione begins circulating in our blood, providing protective glutathione molecules to all organ systems and cells. When delivered in this form, the glutathione is able to enter the cells and provide elevated levels for increased protection. Once in the cell, the higher levels of glutathione are available to the mitochondria, where they help to maintain health and prevent disease.

In *Forever Young,* you are going to learn how to adopt these therapeutic interventions as a means of keeping the mitochondria in a youthful state.

Alpha-Lipoic Acid:
The Universal and Metabolic Antioxidant

Another important antioxidant that can help elevate levels of glutathione in the cell is alpha-lipoic acid (ALA), which has always been important in my research and was first introduced to my readers in *The Wrinkle Cure.* Alpha-lipoic acid is unique as an antioxidant because it is both fat- and water-soluble. This means that it is able to protect all portions of the cell, including the mitochondria. ALA is also a metabolic booster that assists in energy production in the mitochondria. It is found naturally in our cells, locked in an enzyme system that is part of the energy-producing mechanism in the mitochondria.

Just say NO

Another mechanism by which ALA gives protection to the cell and mitochondria is by inhibiting the release of nitric oxide (NO). Free radicals are not alone in acting as a destructive force in the mitochondria; nitric oxide can also wreak havoc (more about this in chapter 2).

Nitric oxide has been studied by thousands of scientists in tens of thousands of laboratories for many years because it has a physiological function. It is a signaling molecule that is important in the central nervous system, arteries, and various cell systems. At elevated levels, NO can have negative effects, especially on mitochondrial function. In fact, nitric oxide plays a key role in the formation and perpetuation of various forms of cancer. **Regulating nitric oxide release has become a new therapeutic strategy being used in the treatment of cancer.** In chapter 2 I will introduce additional substances that can block the production of NO and inflammatory transcription factors.

Increased concentrations of nitric oxide interact with oxygen-free radicals, resulting in the production of a superpotent free radical called *peroxynitrite*. During the metabolic stress seen during sepsis, there is a large release of nitric oxide, which disrupts the electron transport chain within the mitochondria. The powerful antioxidant properties of ALA can inhibit the release of nitric oxide, providing vital protection to the mitochondria. Since ALA is powerful enough to protect the cells during the extreme examples of sepsis and septic shock, it follows that this antioxidant can protect your cells from the changes seen during aging. All of the therapies that protect the mitochondria from damage suffered during sepsis can be implemented to prevent many diseases associated with aging.

ALA also helps with glucose metabolism, which becomes more important as we age. Insulin resistance and the elevated glucose levels of hyperglycemia are rampant in the aging population. Unfortunately, there is an epidemic of insulin resistance, elevated glucose levels, and type 2 diabetes in the young as well, due to poor diet and a sedentary lifestyle. It should come as no surprise that glucose dysregulation is also a hallmark finding in sepsis and in the multiple organ dysfunction system (MODS). ALA helps in the cell's uptake of glucose, independent of the action of insulin. It also sensitizes the insulin receptors in the cell plasma membrane, enabling the cell to utilize insulin and glucose more efficiently. **ALA can help restore blood sugar control and prevent metabolic syndrome and diabetes.**

ALA's powerful antioxidant and anti-inflammatory properties work through several mechanisms. One of the most important is its ability to prevent the activation of pro-inflammatory transcription factors such as NF-κB and AP-1. Once NF-κB is activated in the cytosol (watery portion of the cell) during oxidative stress (excess free radicals), it translocates to the nucleus, where it activates gene expression for the production of pro-inflammatory proteins called cytokines. These include tumor necrosis factor alpha and interleukin-2, -4, and -8. This immune response initiates a cascade of inflammation that interferes with cell function and disrupts mitochondrial energy production, generating even more free radicals.

When ALA is administered in conjunction with NAC, it protects glutathione from destruction and increases glutathione production. ALA is an important tool in preventing cytopathic hypoxia—impaired cellular oxygen use—either acutely in the ICU or chronically in the prevention of aging. When ALA is applied topically, its ability to prevent cell death results in visibly decreased lines and wrinkles, increased skin radiance, and an enhanced overall appearance of the skin.

SS Peptides

Another class of novel mitochondrial antioxidants that play a key role in the treatment of cytopathic hypoxia is the amino acid peptide-based antioxidants. These peptides, which I consider to be one of the most exciting discoveries to date, have been designated the SS (Szeto-Schiller) peptides. As you have learned, protecting the mitochondria is critical in preventing death and disease. Unfortunately, the performance of standard antioxidants has been somewhat disappointing because they have not been able to penetrate the mitochondrial membrane effectively. Without adequate protection, free radicals, both oxygen-based and nitrogen-based, damage the mitochondrial membrane, resulting in impaired function and apoptosis, or cell death.

The discovery of the SS peptides has stimulated tremendous activity among researchers. Some of the research is focused on treating problems in the central nervous system. Thanks to the brain-beauty connection, these peptides are showing great promise for improving the appearance of skin. When applied topically, SS peptides demonstrate significant effectiveness in rejuvenating aging skin.

Beauty: It's Skin Deep

These peptides cannot be administered orally, as the digestive enzymes destroy their therapeutic activity. When placed in my phospholipid carrier system, they rapidly penetrate the skin, greatly improving the clinical appearance of the skin. When they are topically applied, the results are cumulative and continue to accrue with each application. Just some of the benefits include a decrease in fine lines and wrinkles and increased radiance. These effects can be attributed to enhanced energy production in the cells. These visible improvements in the skin can be seen within just a few short weeks of application.

The SS peptides have more than a cosmetic effect. In this carrier system, they are able to penetrate all layers of the skin, reaching the subdermal vasculature, where they enter the bloodstream and circulate throughout the body. Once these peptides enter the cell, they pass through the mitochondrial membrane, giving protection against a variety of highly damaging free radicals. In addition, the SS peptides protect against lipid peroxidation, or fat destruction, providing significant protection to the cell plasma membrane as well as the fragile mitochondrial membrane. These dual actions prevent the cellular damage that occurs during acute sepsis and/or aging. The SS peptides are currently being tested as a treatment for cytopathic hypoxia in the ICU.

Carnitine: A Multifunctional Anti-Inflammatory

Carnitine and its derivative acetyl L-carnitine (ALCAR) are amino acids that are essential in transporting fatty acids into the mitochondria to be burned for energy. Carnitine and ALCAR play a key role in maintaining mitochondrial energy production, which is critical in combating sepsis, MODS, and aging. To ensure that fats will be utilized for energy production in the cell, carnitine levels must be adequate.

Carnitine and ALCAR also protect the mitochondria through an antioxidant mechanism. Carnitine can also decrease the production of pro-inflammatory cytokines such as interleukin-1, interleukin-6, and tumor necrosis factor alpha. The depletion of carnitine results in a highly damaging, systemic inflammatory burst. Since the key to preventing accelerated aging and age-related diseases is controlling inflammation, carnitine and ALCAR are indispensable in achieving this goal.

Since both forms of carnitine aid in transportation of fats into the mitochondria to be used for energy production, they are important in my weight loss regimen described in chapter 3. Carnitine and ALCAR enhance the sensitivity of insulin receptors, helping to decrease blood sugar levels and levels of circulating insulin, necessary to any successful antiaging and weight loss program.

Co Q10

Another important antiaging nutrient that can be used to protect the mitochondria and treat MODS is coenzyme Q10, also known as ubiquinol. Co Q10 is found within the mitochondrial electron transport chain and assists in passing the electrons through the chain for the production of ATP, the energy storage and transfer molecule that is essential to life. Co Q10 is also a powerful antioxidant, used both topically and orally to prevent the clinical and physiological changes seen with aging and aging skin. It has been found effective in reducing the incidence of fine lines and wrinkles in the skin when used orally and/ or topically.

Summary

Although extreme examples, cytopathic hypoxia and MODS can also be a model for aging. Aging is characterized by mitochondrial dysfunction, with a disruption in energy production that eventually leads to cell death by apoptosis. The aging cell is unable to use oxygen even when there is adequate oxygen being delivered to the tissue. Finding therapeutic agents that can protect the mitochondria is critical to all organ systems, including the skin. When these agents are taken orally, there is improved function in all vital organs, including the central nervous system or brain, where they can slow the loss of memory and the decline of problem-solving abilities. They are also critical in preventing the diseases of the cardiovascular system, the greatest cause of mortality in the aging population. When they are applied topically, the results are significant, reducing the classic signs of aging skin, including wrinkles, loss of contour and muscle tone, sagging, loss of radiance, enlarged pores, and discoloration.

You have learned that you can positively affect the way your cells function and you can intervene in the cell death associated with aging.

In chapter 2, I will introduce you to exciting research that will demonstrate that you can manipulate the expression of your genes, turning off disease- and age-accelerating transcription factors and turning on those that fight age and disease. With the tools you will read about in *Forever Young,* you will be able to preserve and restore your vitality and youthful appearance with strategies that are based on the most up-to-date science.

Chapter Two

INTRODUCTION TO NUTRIGENOMICS

A question often posed to me during lectures and public appearances is the following: "Dr. Perricone, isn't it true that genetics play a huge role in my susceptibility to disease and signs of aging?"

Some people ask this question because they want to avoid taking responsibility for their health—assuming that, for good or ill, it is fixed in their genes like their height or their eye color.

As you will discover in this book, this is far from true. We have a great deal more control of our bodies than previously thought. There is an emerging field of study known as nutrigenomics. The word is a combination of *nutrition* and *genomics*. Together, they describe a field that focuses on the relationship between diet and gene expression. Nutrigenomic research investigates questions such as how food influences gene expression and how genes influence the way individuals absorb and metabolize different types of nutrients.

Using nutrigenomics, I will demonstrate how you can actually change the way genes are expressed and how that information is transmitted, simply by manipulating different aspects of your diet and lifestyle. For example, you know that by eating many of the foods included in my anti-inflammatory diet, you can:

1. Switch on protective genes
2. Switch off genes that may have a negative effect on our health

EPIGENETICS
YOU ARE WHAT YOUR GRANDMOTHER ATE!

In addition to altering gene expression with foods and nutrients, you can also alter the epigenome. *Epigenome* is derived from the Greek *epi*, which means "over" or "above," so epigenomes are over and above genes. Epigenome refers to changes in gene expression caused by mechanisms other than changes in the underlying DNA sequence. This is accomplished when molecular tags attach directly to the DNA or to the proteins surrounding the DNA (histones). These molecular tags can be semipermanent and can even be passed on to the next generation.

This means that we can not only change the way our genes are expressed, but change those of our children and perhaps our grandchildren by eating the right foods and obtaining important nutritional factors. The incredibly good health we experience by eating the anti-inflammatory diet can now be conferred on our children and grandchildren. What better gift could we give to our children than the gift of health and vitality? And the good news is that there is no inheritance tax attached.

In this chapter we are going to introduce substances that turn *off* disease and age-accelerating transcription factors such as NF-κB and AP-1 and turn *on* the age- and disease-fighting transcription factor NRF2. This not inconsiderable feat is accomplished by a class of exotic-sounding substances known as *Michael acceptor pharmacophores.* This process is one of the most fascinating and exciting aspects of my research during the past decade. The remarkably protective properties of Michael acceptor pharmacophores are one of our finest strategies for staying Forever Young. In addition, I will introduce you to phytonutrients with other pharmacophores, which act as powerful anti-inflammatories through similar mechanisms.

In many of my books, I have discussed transcription factors, the protein messengers in our cells that are activated or silenced by different stimuli. Upon activation, these transcription factors translocate to the nucleus of the cell, where they attach to receptor sites on the genes and upregulate, or turn on, their expression. Gene expression provides us with a new strategy to suppress pro-inflammatory genes. This is critical because, as you know, inflammation is the common denominator of all the problems we see with aging and age-related disease.

But research has shown us that it is not just the transcription factors that play a role in gene expression; we now know that nutrients can also affect gene expression in many ways. **My research has revealed a number of novel compounds, naturally found in our diet, that can powerfully and positively affect gene expression.**

When these nutrients upregulate gene expression, the following benefits result:

- Healthy body weight
- Resistance to cognitive decline
- Decreased incidence of cancer
- Prevention and reversal of insulin resistance and metabolic syndrome
- Maintenance of bone density

- Optimal function of all vital organs, including the heart, kidney, spleen, and immune system
- Maintenance of muscle mass
- Well-functioning endocrine system that keeps us fit and sexually active into our later years
- Prevention and reduction of damage to the skin caused by aging and the environment

These lofty claims may sound unrealistic, but when it comes to nutrigenomics, the results are well documented.

Living Life to the Max

When scientists study longevity, they consider two parameters. The first is the *average* life span of a species, which in humans in the United States is about 78.2 years. The second is the *maximum* life span, the longest a member of that species has lived, which has remained at about 115 to 120 calendar years throughout recorded history, despite steady improvements in life expectancy. The longest unambiguously documented life span is that of Jeanne Calment of France (1875–1997), who died at age 122 years, 164 days.

When I first began studying the aging process several decades ago, I looked at various aging theories and interventions. At that time, there were no pharmacological therapies that could increase the maximum life span.

Many agents increased the average life span in animals, but maximum human life span extension appeared out of reach. A breakthrough came with the introduction of caloric restriction (CR). CR is one of the few documented dietary interventions that have been found to increase both the median and the maximum life span in a variety of species, among them yeast, fish, rodents, and dogs. Rats, mice, and hamsters, for example, experience better health and maximum life-span extension from a normal diet that contains 40 to 60 percent of the calories, but all of the required nutrients, that the animals consume when they can eat as much as they want.

CR studies have not been done with primates or humans because of the complexity of the cells and organ systems. We do not know if it would work. As I have told my patients, if you can force yourself to eat 60 percent less on a daily basis, you may not live to be 150, but it will seem that way.

Science has now discovered that the mechanism of life extension seen in CR results from the activation of a gene group affecting multiple factors that prolong life. Some of the factors regulated by this gene pool are:

- Blood glucose levels
- Lipid profiles
- Muscle mass
- Cognitive function
- Overall control of oxidative stress in the cells

We now know that CR activates protective genes and at the same time prevents the expression of negative genes that can result in cancer, diabetes, and obesity.

In this chapter, I am going to introduce some newer substances that I have been working with that promise to deliver many of the benefits of CR without its hardships and limitations.

One such substance is the phytonutrient resveratrol, the antioxidant found in red grapes and red wine. Resveratrol is the best-known member of a family of compounds called stilbenes, the general name for which is stilbene synthase (STS). Scientists are studying resveratrol because it seems to help express the same genes that are expressed during caloric restriction.

Activating the Longevity Factors

Thanks to my appearances on public television, *Oprah*, *GMA*, the *Today* show, and other popular venues, many people refer to me as the "Salmon and Blueberry Doctor." It is true that wild salmon and blueberries held center stage in my first book, *The Wrinkle Cure*, in which I introduced the anti-inflammatory diet. There are many reasons for this. Salmon and the other cold-water fish are an outstanding source of high-quality protein; carotenoid antioxidants, like astaxanthin, which you will read about in chapter 4; and high levels of the omega-3s and other essential fats, all of which have powerful anti-inflammatory effects.

Roses Are Red, Violets Are Blue
(Thanks to the Anthocyanins)

Blueberries are also antioxidant powerhouses containing a variety of phytonutrients, including anthocyanins, from the Greek *anthos*, meaning "flower" plus *kyanos*, meaning "blue." Anthocyanins may be the most important of the visible plant pigments, responsible for the reds, purples, and blues you see in plants that have strong antioxidant properties. They are found in such fruits as blueberries, blackberries, raspberries, black raspberries, black currants, açai, and chokeberry and vegetables including red cabbage, watercress, and eggplant. Anthocyanins provide many different functions for the plant. They are antioxidants, protect the plant against UV light, are a defense mechanism, and have an important role in pollination and reproduction. The purple pansy, for example, owes its color to anthocyanins, which attract insects to propagate the species.

As antioxidants, anthocyanins protect plants from free radicals produced by sunlight or damage to the plant. The ability of the anthocyanins to protect plants from free-radical damage can also benefit us when we eat foods that are rich in anthocyanins.

As mentioned earlier in this chapter, blueberries contain many powerful polyphenols that make them a true superfood, one that I have been recommending for decades. We know that they are rich in polyphenols such as the anthocyanins, which have many benefits, including the following.

- They have the ability to speed up neural communication. Blueberry-supplemented neurons have a better ability to communicate with each other.
- Catechins contained in blueberries prevent cell death and the loss of nerve growth factors.
- Blueberries increase the release of dopamine, an energizing, stimulatory neurotransmitter.
- Blueberries protect us from age-associated declines in dopamine levels, helping us to maintain youthful brain function.

Anthocyanins also possess a special form of stilbenes known as *pterostilbene*, which activates the genes that influence longevity factors. This is another reason choosing brightly colored fruits and vegetables is essential. The colors signify the presence of plant pigments, which do more than just add color to fruits, vegetables, and certain seafood. **Colorful fruits and vegetables serve as the top dietary sources of disease-preventive phytonutrients and antiaging antioxidants.** But, this is not the entire story. We now know that many of these phytonutrients also work through other mechanisms, specifically the expression of genes that can upregulate the natural protective mechanisms of our cells.

Superfoods and Spices for Beautiful Skin

I believe that foods have an extremely powerful effect on our physical and mental well-being. **Functioning very much like pharmacologi-**

cal agents, foods can dramatically alter the biochemistry of cells, affecting both cell and organ function. Food is what provides the body with the nutrients needed for cellular growth and repair. As we age, cellular inflammation disrupts the cell's normal biochemical functions, negatively affecting all organ systems. We know that the high-glycemic carbohydrates—sugars and starches—cause a rapid rise in blood sugar and insulin and generate an inflammatory response. In addition, synthetic foods like trans fats and other chemical additives disrupt cellular function by either increasing inflammation or functioning as toxins.

Inflammation and the Skin

The skin is eventually damaged by this chronic low-grade inflammation, which manifests in the classic signs of aging, including wrinkling, sagging, discoloration, enlarged pores, and lack of radiance. We long for a radiant, youthful complexion and try unsuccessfully to achieve this with a variety of cosmetics and potions that offer "hope in a jar" and not much else.

But there is good news. It has been shown that after only three days of the anti-inflammatory diet, skin looks significantly healthier, more radiant, and less wrinkled. And topical anti-inflammatories, many of them from food-sourced antioxidants, provide many visible benefits. We are now ready for the next generation of topical therapies, which rely on nutrigenomics and the marvel of gene expression.

Designer Genes for Flawless Skin

Food-based nutrients can alter gene expression. As a dermatologist, I have been delighted to learn that when these nutrients are applied topically, they can upregulate the expression of genes that decrease and/or

THE RAINBOW FOODS—
COLOR IS THE KEY TO GENE EXPRESSION

I have long encouraged my patients to shop for the "rainbow foods" in the produce aisle. A full palette of sensual color will not only make your food beautiful, it will heal your body on a cellular level and will keep you young. Choose from the array of fresh fruits and vegetables at the market or, even better, at a local farmers' market:

- A variety of baby greens, including watercress and arugula
- Red cabbage
- Dark green broccoli, broccoli rabe, broccolini
- String beans
- Red onions and tomatoes
- Purple garlic
- Red, purple, and yellow bell peppers
- Bright red chile peppers
- Purple eggplant
- Alfalfa and broccoli sprouts
- Fragrant fresh herbs and spices, including basil, parsley, thyme, rosemary, sage, oregano, dill, cinnamon sticks, golden turmeric root, thyme
- Deep blue blueberries
- Brilliant blackberries
- Vivid red strawberries
- Royal purple plums
- Deep red or bright green apples
- Red-black Bing cherries

For condiments:

- Dark green extra-virgin olive oil
- An assortment of green and black olives

In the bulk food department, stock up on:

- Dark red kidney beans
- Black and red lentils
- Golden oats
- Warm brown walnuts
- Dark chocolate
- Almonds
- Bright green pumpkin seeds

And don't forget seafood:

- Rich, red Alaskan sockeye salmon
- Maine lobster
- Deep pink Alaskan king crab legs
- Shrimp

For even more on the rainbow foods, see chapter 8, "The Forever Young Kitchen and Recipes."

---

prevent inflammation. By assisting the cells' normal ability to repair themselves, these nutrients produce a more youthful appearance with positive, visible changes in a matter of days.

Messengers

All antioxidants act as anti-inflammatories, but not all phytonutrients are necessarily antioxidants. There are other important factors at work. Although antioxidants are an important part of the picture, the antioxidant hypothesis is an oversimplification of the biochemical story. Antioxidants do neutralize free radicals, but we now know that they do much more. Both antioxidants and phytonutrients have the power to alter the genetic instructions found in our genes' DNA, which holds our genetic blueprint. Antioxidants and other nutrients can also act as *signaling* mechanisms in the cell. By means of gene expression, they upregulate the cell's natural protective and regulatory functions, which then promote the visible differences that we are searching for.

Seeing Blue and Going Green: Nutrigenomics in Action

The nutrients and other substances discussed in this chapter provide benefits that far exceed their function as antioxidants. Green, black, and white tea (*Camellia sinensis*), cocoa, and blueberries all contain special catechins (with active pharmacophores) that have significant effects on gene expression.

Tea has many benefits and is well known for both its anticancer and its antioxidant properties. Other positive effects include:

- The amino acid called theonine, a natural relaxant that won't make you drowsy
- The ability to increase metabolism, resulting in the burning of body fat
- The ability to suppress the absorption of fat
- High levels of antioxidants that act as anti-inflammatories and are protective for the skin and brain, and all your organs
- The ability to improve glucose tolerance in diabetic mice, an effect that may help prevent type 2 diabetes
- High levels of an important polyphenol antioxidant, epigallocatechin gallate (EGCG), which is believed to be responsible for much of green tea's promise in the prevention of cardiovascular disease, obesity, Alzheimer's disease, cancer, periodontal disease, and dental cavities

- Topical application of low-dose green tea extract may help protect against UV damage, without the common side effects

What I find so exciting about substances like EGCG and related catechins is their ability to bind to the signaling molecules that either *block* or *activate* transcription factors. In other words, the EGCG found in tea can inhibit the activation of NF-κB, thereby blocking all of the pro-inflammatory cytokines normally generated when it is activated. The EGCG may also bind to the protective transcription factor NRF2, upregulating many of our antioxidant defense systems.

Beyond Antioxidants

Although the antioxidant activity of many of these substances may have a minor role in their protection against cancer, heart disease, Alzheimer's disease, and wrinkles, it is not the main reason for their outstanding antiaging, chemoprotective properties. Their mild *pro-oxidant* effects are the real heroes, because they *activate* protective transcription factors such as NRF2 as they *inhibit* damaging transcription factors such as NF-κB.

For example, we have known for years that blueberries improved memory and protected the skin, but it was not until the discovery of nutrigenomics that I learned their elusive mechanism of action, which can be attributed to the presence of the catechins. As with all of the substances discussed in this chapter, this mechanism of action *exceeds* their status as antioxidants. Their pro-oxidant activity results in the production of more than fifteen or twenty cell-protective enzymes that are produced by the activation of the genes controlled by transcription factors.

At the same time, the molecules that we thought were *just* antioxidants bind to and turn off transcription factors that are known to upregulate more than a hundred inflammation-generating genes, resulting in damage to all of our organ systems. For example, when activated, age-accelerating transcription factors produce a host of pro-inflammatory cytokines that can drive the formation of cancer. At the same time, the cell's ability to turn on apoptosis (programmed cell death) is turned off. In other words, age-accelerating transcription factors prevent cancer cells from self-destruction. When the activation of these transcription factors is blocked, all of their cancer-promoting properties are turned off and apoptosis, which results in the self-destruction of the cancer cells, is turned on. **All of the substances you will read about in this chapter have the ability to deactivate age-accelerating transcription factors and to activate the protective transcription factor.**

Catechins such as EGCG act like Michael acceptor pharmacophores, controlling gene expression by binding with the thiols in these transcription factors. Once again, the nutrigenomic aspect of dietary substances proves to be the mechanism of action that far exceeds their antioxidant capabilities. Scientists still do not understand the significance of the sulfur-binding capability of EGCG and the other catechins, which allows them to control the very powerful transcription factors for good or ill.

WRINKLE BLOCKER

The EGCG in tea prevents the activation of collagen-digesting enzymes known as matrix metalloproteinase. This is a critical function because these enzymes are responsible for wrinkling of the skin.

Blueberries, cocoa, and tea, with active pharmacophores, are perfect examples of how nutritional factors exert control of gene expression. A pharmacophore is a set of structural features in a molecule that is recognized at a receptor site. This set of features is responsible for the molecule's biological activity. Nutrigenomics, the common factor and theme throughout this book, clarifies, for the first time, the previously unknown mechanism of action of these food substances.

The Future Is Now

Scientists working on the Human Genome Project talk of a bright future for genetic manipulation, one that will someday change our lives for the better. But I am telling you that right now, today, the rainbow foods that are gracing our dinner tables in all of their colorful, flavorful, and aromatic glory hold the key to turning on the protective, restorative genes and turning off the damaging ones. As might be expected, pro-inflammatory foods turn off the protective genes and turn on the damaging ones. As children we can get away with quite a bit and not have it show up on our face or body. However, as we age, our bodies are not so forgiving, and pro-inflammatory foods are manifested in a very visible manner: puffy eyes, wrinkled, sagging skin, enlarged pores, discolorations, dullness, acne, loss of youthful contours, and so forth.

Some nutrients pack a powerful nutrigenomic punch with many benefits. This chapter will examine the beneficial effects of watercress; essential fatty acids; cinnamon, turmeric, and other spices; chocolate; and vitamin D.

In addition, you will learn about new research on free radicals that uses *spin traps,* molecules that are able to catch volatile free radicals so that they can be studied.

Nitroalkenes, the Miracle of Modified Essential and Unsaturated Fatty Acids

The human body has many complex pathways for regulating biochemical functions, including inflammation, which is necessary for an immune response. As you well know, inflammation results in tissue destruction and ultimately death when unabated.

In chapter 1, I introduced the concept of cytopathic hypoxia, which is seen in acute sepsis and septic shock, as a model for accelerated aging. The multiple organ dysfunction syndrome (MODS) that I became familiar with in the ICU as a medical student and resident was an unforgettable experience. Now, recent research illustrates the intelligence of the cell and how the body can outwit the enemy on the twin battlefields of aging and disease.

The lung is one of the vital organs affected in septic shock. Pulmonary inflammation with multiple complications can lead to death. The designation for this group of respiratory symptoms is known as acute respiratory distress syndrome (ARDS), which is caused on a cellular level by the release of multiple pro-inflammatory cytokines.

The cytokines, including tumor necrosis factor alpha and interleukin-1, -4, -6, -8, and -10, result in a cascade of events that are highly destructive to lung tissue. The inflammatory cascade induces the release of nitric oxide (NO). A chemical messenger, NO, is needed for cell communication and for the relaxation of blood vessels, among many physiological functions. Unfortunately, with ARDS, excessive amounts of NO are released. This increases free-radical production and cytokine formation, resulting in pulmonary edema, or water on the lungs. Pulmonary edema can be a chronic condition, or it can develop suddenly, as in the case of septic shock, when it quickly becomes life threatening. This life-threatening pulmonary edema occurs when a large amount of fluid suddenly shifts from the pulmonary blood vessels into the lung due to lung problems, heart attack, trauma, or toxic chemicals.

Linoleic Acid to the Rescue

Though ARDS may seem like an extreme example, I have chosen it because it so beautifully describes the intelligence of the cell and the body's innate powers to heal itself. Through the incredible complexity of cell function, the excess nitric oxide released in ARDS begins chemically combining with the essential fatty acid linoleic acid. This omega-6 unsaturated fatty acid is essential to cell function and in this instance acts as a natural therapeutic compound. Once linoleic acid combines with the nitrogen at one of its double bonds, a substance known as nitrolinoleic acid (LNO_2) is formed. This newly created signaling molecule rapidly starts turning down the inflammation and counteracting the effects of the pro-inflammatory cytokines.

The Intelligent Cell in Action—Nitro Fatty Acids (Nitroalkenes)

In the face of powerful inflammatory chemicals like nitric oxide, the cell mounts a stunning defense: it provides an essential fatty acid, which then combines with the offensive agent to make an antidote that counteracts its negative effects. The effects of nitrolinoleic acid on cell mechanisms are currently generating great interest in the scientific world.

This anti-inflammatory signaling agent upregulates the expression of a gene that encodes for a cell-protective substance called heme oxygenase 1 (HO-1). HO-1 is a cell-protective enzyme that falls under the classification of heat-shock proteins. Heat-shock proteins give the cell great resistance to inflammation and other stressors such as hyperthermia, abnormally high body temperature. HO-1 also confers protection in chronic inflammatory diseases like rheumatoid arthritis and other autoimmune problems.

As exciting as these particular discoveries are, the upregulation of the production of HO-1 is just one of many ways that nitrolinoleic acid provides protection to our bodies. Continued research has revealed that very low concentrations of nitrolinoleic acid inhibit the expression of various pro-inflammatory genes, blocking the production of cytokines and cytokine receptors. The most exciting action of nitrolinoleic acid, in my opinion, is the upregulation of NRF2, which, as you know, is hugely important, as it protects cells from oxidative stress (free-radical damage and subsequent inflammation). It works by upregulating the expression of cell-protective genes, including those that produce glutathione, the cells' chief antioxidant. Once glutathione is increased, it begins one of its many cell-protective functions such as scooping up oxygen- or nitrogen-based free radicals. It also protects against inflammation by inhibiting the pro-inflammatory transcription factors such as NF-κB and AP-1. Because it inhibits the activation of NF-κB, excess production of cell-damaging nitric oxide is also blocked. This is a critical function of glutathione, because chronically elevated levels of NO can lead to tumor formation.

Glutathione acts as a cofactor for other antioxidant enzymes. These include glutaredoxins and the glutathione S-transferases. This powerful antioxidant also regenerates the water-soluble antioxidant vitamin C, which then interacts with the fat-soluble vitamin E and Co Q10, helping to keep the antioxidant levels of those intact.

Nitrolinoleic acid has proved to be protective of several vital organ systems and also neuroprotective, guarding our nervous system from the damage that can lead to Alzheimer's or Parkinson's disease. As we learned in the brain/beauty connection, what is good for the brain is also therapeutic for the skin. I am predicting that the nitrofatty acids will be very useful when applied topically to the skin for treatment of the clinical changes in aging skin.

Scientists anticipate that nitrolinoleic acid supplements will confer many systemic benefits, including the prevention of hypertension (high blood pressure), diabetes, and stroke, and promoting healthy weight loss. Weight loss is a particularly fascinating aspect of the action of nitrolinoleic acid. Like the omega-3 essential fatty acids, nitrolinoleic acid activates nuclear receptors known as *peroxisome proliferator-activated receptors,* or PPARs. These receptors, located in the cell nucleus, control blood sugar levels, the storing and burning of body fat, and the way energy is used in the body. It appears that nitrolinoleic acid strongly binds to and activates PPARs, providing significant protection against the high blood sugar associated with type 2 diabetes while dramatically reducing excess body fat.

Nitroalkenes (Chemistry)

Cellular chemistry is complex and elegant. Some mild oxidizing agents or electrophiles can have beneficial effects on cellular health. These mild electrophiles are the active constituents found in watercress and the spices cinnamon and turmeric, and unique substances known as *spin traps* and nitroalkenes. These mild electrophiles, also known as Michael acceptor pharmacophores, and other similarly acting pharmacophores are of tremendous importance in the dual battlefields of aging and disease.

Crying Wolf

As we know, nitroalkenes are slightly electrophilic or mild oxidizing agents. Through what would normally be perceived as a negative action, they exert positive effects on the cell. Whenever I observe a nitrogen molecule adjacent to a carbon molecule with a double bond, I am reminded that nitrogen tends to pull electrons away, making the carbon electron-deficient. If a molecule is electron-deficient, it becomes electron-hungry, or electrophilic, and can now be looked upon as an oxidizing agent. As in the case of nitroalkenes and the spices and spin traps I will discuss later in this chapter, this is a mild effect that is not detrimental to the cell structure; however, it is strong enough to trick the protective transcription factor NRF2 into thinking that there is severe

TURNING UP THE HEAT TO BURN BODY FAT

When I was young, I could eat as much as I wanted and not gain any weight. My body would throw off a tremendous amount of body heat after a meal. This process is known as *postprandial thermogenesis,* which means the production of heat after eating. It is no coincidence that overweight people have very little postprandial thermogenesis. I noticed that as I got older, I started to put on weight; at the same time, the amount of heat my body dissipated after a meal decreased significantly. I began a quest to understand what was happening on a biochemical level.

Breaking Up Is Hard to Do

I learned that food calories can be burned in the mitochondria for production of adenosine triphosphate (ATP), a high-energy phosphate molecule used to store and release energy for work within the body. This entire process is known as *oxidative phosphorylation.*

Food can be stored as body fat (triglycerides in adipose tissue) or stored as glycogen in the liver and muscles. Glycogen is the form in which foods are stored in the body as energy. If we can "uncouple" the oxidation from the phosphorylation, food calories can be burned off by thermogenesis.

Thermogenesis (body heat) bypasses the ATP-mediated energy. **If the majority of the food we eat can be transformed into body heat, we stay thin with low body fat stores.**

When I entered medical school, I was searching for a natural agent to uncouple the oxidation from the phosphorylation as a possible strategy for weight loss. Unfortunately, the uncoupling agents that I found were toxic—but I never gave up trying.

Eventually I found that essential fatty acids, such as the omega-3s found in fish oil, chia seeds, and cold-water fish such as salmon and sardines, could uncouple oxidative phosphorylation. They do this through the PPARs discussed above, which partition energy so that it is not stored as fat. They also downregulate enzymes that synthesize fat. Thus, essential fatty acids can affect gene expression by activating PPARs that turn on the fat-burning genes.

Omega-3s produce a protein known as *uncoupling protein 3*, which uncouples oxidative phosphorylation. This results in more energy being dissipated as heat and a decrease in stored body fat. As we have learned, the nitroalkenes—nitrolinoleic acid, for example—strongly bind to and activate the PPARs, resulting in even greater weight loss, partitioning of energy, and uncoupling of oxidative phosphorylation. For more weight loss strategies including a discussion of omega 3–rich chia seeds, see chapter 3, "The Metabolic Miracle."

---

oxidative stress present. In response to this "threat," NRF2 moves to the nucleus and activates multiple cell-protective genes to come to the rescue.

But that's not all. In addition to activating the good guys, mild electrophiles like the nitroalkenes, the curcuminoids found in turmeric, active constituents of watercress and cinnamon and the spin traps, deactivate the bad guys, just as we observed with the catechins found in blueberries, cocoa, and tea. They do this through the same mechanism that inhibits the activation of the pro-inflammatory transcription factor NF-κB. They work their positive effects by acting as electrophilic Michael acceptors, which activate good transcription factors such as NRF2. At the same time, they inhibit NF-κB and other pro-inflammatory transcription factors. The net effect is extremely beneficial: control of inflammation throughout our cells and organ systems, both in aging and in acute disease.

The Old-New Superfoods—Cinnamon and Turmeric: Spices of Life

NRF2 to the rescue

Cinnamon is not only a delicious spice, it has a variety of health benefits, starting with one of the keys to staying Forever Young and wrinkle-free, the regulation of blood sugar.

The USDA Human Nutrition Research Center in Beltsville, Maryland, is a world leader in research on the links between nutrition and disease. In one study, the scientists were amazed to find that volunteers who had eaten apple pie, high in sugar and refined flour, did not experience the expected large rise in their blood sugar levels.

They soon discovered that cinnamon, that wonderfully fragrant, classic apple pie spice, was the reason. Cinnamon contains a variety of phytonutrients, including the flavan-3-ol polyphenol-class antioxidants similar to those found in grapes, berries, cocoa, and green tea (OPCs and catechins).

This class of antioxidants boosts the stabilizing effect of insulin on blood sugar. At the same time, these antioxidants inhibit insulin resistance. They achieve this by activating enzymes that stimulate insulin receptors, making the cells more sensitive to insulin, increasing insulin's ability to lower blood sugar. In addition, they augment the effects of the insulin-signaling pathways within skeletal muscle tissue.

Just a few of the benefits of these phytonutrients are as follows:

- Cinnamon acts as a powerful anti-inflammatory. It inhibits the release of the inflammatory fatty acid arachidonic acid from platelet membranes. It also reduces the production of an inflammatory prostaglandin (messenger) called thromboxane A2.
- Its essential oil inhibits the growth of bacteria and fungi.
- It functions as a strong antioxidant.

- Its strong, fragrant aroma boosts cognitive processing in the brain, improving memory and attention span.

Barking Up the Right Tree

The essential oil that is extracted from *Cinnamomum cassia* bark is one of the core spice derivatives in the miracle of gene expression. Cinnamon has many activities, as described, and its powerful antioxidant properties protect and enhance many cellular functions that promote health and longevity. Cinnamon is also a powerful antimicrobial, which means it can fight infections in the body and help the immune system stave off infectious disease. Cinnamon also has a tremendous ability to act as an antipyretic, reducing fever in a manner similar to aspirin or Tylenol, without the negative side effects. The antidiabetic activities of cinnamon have been researched and discussed in many of my previous books and lectures. Cinnamon's ability to stabilize blood sugar levels and prevent a subsequent insulin response is a powerful tool, one that can be used on a daily basis to prevent spikes in blood sugar levels. It is these fluctuations in blood sugar that are one of the primary causes of chronic subclinical inflammation and weight gain. Many of cinnamon's activities have been attributed to the antioxidants present, such as the proanthocyanidins, but further research has revealed that the antioxidant/free-radical paradigm is simplistic and somewhat inaccurate.

The Cloud with the Silver Lining

Cinnamon contains a key flavor compound known as cinnamic aldehyde. This compound is extracted and used for flavoring candy, toothpaste, and mouthwash. Most of us are familiar with this delicious and somewhat spicy flavor and aroma. This flavoring agent has a slight ability to steal electrons very much like that of the free radicals. Like the nitroalkenes, it is classified as a Michael acceptor. Normally, you would think that this was not a good thing, but this cloud has a silver lining.

This ability to attract electrons has earned cinnamic aldehyde its electrophile classification, but cinnamic aldehyde has mild or weak activity. We know that transcription factors can be activated by oxidative stress. When cinnamic aldehyde, a weak electrophile, acts upon NRF2, this protective transcription factor is activated, just as it is when a cell is under attack by free radicals. Now activated, NRF2 moves to the nucleus of the cell and attaches to the genes that produce multiple protective, anti-inflammatory enzymes. As this protective set of genes is unleashed, the cell becomes flooded with antioxidant enzymes and anti-inflammatories.

Finding substances that can turn on the highly protective transcription factor NRF2 holds the key to preventing a host of diseases. When phytonutrients and other molecules that contain the Michael acceptor–like pharmacophore upregulate the transcription factor NRF2, more than a dozen protective anti-inflammatory proteins in the cell are activated. These cell-protective proteins are referred to as phase 2 protective proteins. When this natural cell-protective mechanism is achieved with phytonutrients, the response is far superior to the protective action of antioxidants alone, because such antioxidants as vitamin C and Co Q10 are consumed when neutralizing free radicals. Phytonutrients act as catalysts and the action on gene expression is indirect. Instead of being consumed by the free radicals, the phytonutrients can provide long-term protection to the cell.

Derivatives of cinnamic aldehyde can now be used to protect cells from carcinogenic and other toxic agents. When applied topically, they give skin cells tremendous protection from environmental stressors—ultraviolet light from excessive sun exposure, for example—as well as other environmental pro-inflammatory agents. Topically applied derivatives of cinnamic aldehyde, both before and after sunburn, can rescue the cells and prevent them from turning precancerous. Topical application also prevents the apoptosis, or cell death, associated with sunburn. Skin cells damaged by ultraviolet radiation are the extreme end of the inflammation spectrum. Since derivatives of cinnamic aldehyde have the ability to protect even severely damaged cells, they are highly effective as a topical antiaging agent that can be used on a daily basis. It is important to note that *derivatives* of cinnamic aldehyde, not cinnamic aldehyde itself, are used. This distinction is significant, because cinnamic aldehyde is a sensitizing agent and can create both irritation and an allergic reaction when applied to the skin.

Stopping a Deadly Cancer

One of the most exciting developments in the use of the cinnamic aldehyde Michael acceptor is its efficacy in the treatment of the deadly cancer melanoma. I have seen many patients present with an abnormal-looking mole, a pigmented lesion, on their skin that proved to be melanoma when biopsied. This dreaded diagnosis is not something you ever want to see. When I am doing a biopsy and suspect the worst, I hope that the melanoma has not gone very deep, because if it has grown unchecked, the cancer then metastasizes to other organ systems, reducing life expectancy to less than a year for these poor unsuspecting patients.

If the lesion is identified early enough, a surgical excision with a wide margin around the lesion is curative. Unfortunately, metastatic melanoma is extremely aggressive and very resistant to existing chemotherapeutic regimens. There is a great need for a pharmacologic agent that will be effective in the treatment of this deadly cancer.

With cinnamic aldehyde, it now looks as if we may have the answer. When scientists tested cinnamic aldehyde against human melanoma cells in a cell culture system and also in animal models, it showed efficacy against this deadly cancer. An important study by Christopher Cabello and his colleagues at the Department of Pharmacology and Toxicology, College of Pharmacy, Arizona Cancer Center, University of Arizona, Tucson, concludes that **cinnamic aldehyde shows exceptional promise in both the prevention and the treatment of melanoma.** I am currently working with colleagues to begin a human study with this remarkable substance.

Turmeric—Worth Its Weight in Gold

Turmeric is another spice containing the Michael acceptors. We are all familiar with this delicious spice, the hallmark of fragrant, flavorful golden curries.

Curcumin, chemically diferuloylmethane, and its derivatives demethoxycurcumin and bisdemethoxycurcumin, collectively known as curcuminoids, are responsible for the yellow pigment derived from the roots of the perennial herb turmeric (*Curcuma longa L.*). They are also responsible for turmeric's exceptional health-promoting properties. The curcuminoids prevent NF-κB from activation with extreme efficiency.

In fact, the single most promising food-derived compound to combat cancer, based on the current body of scientific evidence, is the curcuminoids found in turmeric. M. D. Anderson Hospital in Houston, Texas, and other top cancer research centers in the United States are involved in preclinical and clinical research on the anticancer mechanism and application of curcuminoids in conditions including colon, breast, head, neck, and prostate cancer, multiple myeloma, and respiratory tract cancers. The curcuminoids prevent NF-κB activation with extreme efficiency.

Many studies indicate that turmeric in general, and its curcuminoid fraction specifically, possess significant potential in preventing and treating cancer. The active constituents in turmeric have tremendous activity in the body, protecting several organ systems including the brain and heart.

The curcuminoids found in turmeric also function as a mild electrophile or Michael acceptor. By acting as a mild oxidizing agent, they activate the protective transcription factor NRF2, which then upregulates a multitude of cell-protective enzymes and molecules. Scientists are now studying the protective effects of NRF2 activation in reducing oxidative stress found in the central nervous system in diseases such as Alzheimer's, Parkinson's, and Huntington's. **Ingesting turmeric root**

on a daily basis can help prevent the loss of cognitive function that we face as we age.

As predicted by the brain/beauty hypothesis, the curcuminoids found in turmeric are also active in the skin. When applied topically, they function as a powerful anti-inflammatory agent, partially because of their ability to upregulate NRF2, which provides the skin with many benefits, including increased radiance, decreased pore size, and, with continued use, a reduction in fine lines and discolorations.

The Antioxidant Attributes of Turmeric

- The curcuminoid pigments in turmeric are safe, highly effective antioxidants.
- Turmeric turmerin, a unique peptide, acts as a free-radical scavenger and offers 80 percent protection against oxidative injury to membranes and DNA.
- Animals fed curcuminoids show higher blood levels of the enzyme glutathione S-transferase, which, as we learned in chapter 1, is essential to our health as an important antioxidant and key player in the body's detoxification system.

The Anti-inflammatory Powers of Turmeric

- By modulating the effects of key pro-inflammatory molecules, including cyclooxygenase 2, leukotrienes, prostaglandins, nitric oxide, interferon-inducible protein, tumor necrosis factor (TNF), and interleukin-12, the curcuminoids in turmeric suppress inflammation.
- Like alpha-lipoic acid (ALA), curcumin inhibits the proinflammatory actions of nuclear factor kappa-B (NF-κB) and activator protein 1 (AP-1). As you will learn in "The Birth of a Wrinkle," on page 60, activation of NF-κB and AP-1 leads to inflammation-related microscarring of collagen, resulting in wrinkles.

- The curcuminoids may enhance the secretion of anti-inflammatory corticosteroids from the adrenal glands or boost their anti-inflammatory power.
- The curcuminoids are safer anti-inflammatory agents than the standard NSAIDs such as aspirin and ibuprofen. They work by blocking the pro-inflammatory mediator thromboxane (TXA-2) and not by blocking COX-1, which can result in gastric bleeding.
- Turmeric sensitizes the body's cortisol receptor sites, which is important as we age, as elevated cortisol damages all organ systems, including skin.

Eliminating Liver Toxins

When we ingest turmeric, it increases the liver's ability to eliminate dangerous carcinogenic toxins. Studies indicate that it raises the levels of two key liver detoxification enzymes (UDP glucoronyl transferase and glutathione S-transferase).

Spice Up Your Life

Many spice-derived phytochemicals have important therapeutic effects, including their ability to suppress NF-κB. The bad news is that once NF-κB is activated, it induces the expression of more than two hundred genes. As you have learned in these pages, NF-κB is linked to many diseases, including:

AIDS	Cancer
Allergy	Crohn's disease
Alzheimer's disease	Diabetes
Arthritis	Multiple sclerosis
Atherosclerosis	Myocardial infarction

Obesity   Septic shock
Psoriasis

The good news is that many popular foods and spices found in every good cook's kitchen can come to the rescue and suppress this diabolical transcription factor. That NF-κB has been linked to this wide variety of diseases is not too surprising because most diseases are caused by dysregulated inflammation. Thus, agents that can suppress NF-κB activation, in principle, have the potential to prevent or delay the onset of or treat NF-κB-linked diseases.

Phytochemicals in Spices That Suppress NF-κB

Basil, rosemary (ursolic acid)
Blueberries (catechins)
Cinnamon (cinnamic aldehyde)
Cloves (eugenol, isoeugenol)
Cocoa (catechins)
Fennel, anise, coriander (anethol)
Garlic (diallyl sulfide, ajoene, S-allyl cysteine, allicin)
Ginger (6-gingerol)
Green tea (catechins, especially epigallocatechin [EGCG])
Pomegranate (ellagic acid)
Red chiles (capsaicin)
Turmeric (curcumin)

A majority of the active phytochemicals found in spices have antioxidant and anti-inflammatory activities. S. Shobana and K. A. Naidu and their colleagues examined the antioxidant activities of commonly used spices, including garlic, ginger, onion, mint, cloves, cinnamon, and pepper. Among the spices tested, cloves exhibited the greatest antioxidant activity. As we are learning, thanks to nutrigenomics, antioxidant activity is only part of the story. Another part is the ability of these substances to mimic oxidative stress, thus tricking the protective transcription factors into action.

Watercress: An Extraordinary Superfood

One of my great joys in researching and writing this book has been discovering "new" superfoods. And though they may be new to many readers, they are in fact ancient, known throughout history for remarkable healing and rejuvenating properties yet all but forgotten in today's world of fast and processed "food."

Watercress is a case in point. In our modern times, this green is relegated to serving as a garnish or as a tea party staple in the form of wimpy sandwiches cut into fancy shapes. Unfortunately, the vast majority of people do not realize the role of watercress in keeping us Forever Young, which I hope to remedy in this chapter. Watercress, like the spices and green tea, contains the active pharmacophores that control transcription factors and gene expression.

Veggie Tales

I recently had the opportunity to meet with Richard Burgoon, the president and owner, and Andy Brown, the vice president of marketing, of B&W Quality Growers, the world's largest grower and shipper of cultivated watercress. Its founding family has celebrated 140 years as watercress farmers.

Though I have long known of the tremendous health and longevity benefits of the cruciferous vegetables, I was truly amazed to learn about the remarkable nutrient-rich properties of watercress. On a tour of one of B&W's wonderful farms, Richard explained to me that watercress is extremely perishable and a challenge to grow, requiring the perfect combination of pure and cold water, ideal weather conditions, and unique soil requirements. To provide for a consistent year-round supply, B&W has developed a unique network of smaller sustainable seasonal farms in six states. This "follow-the-sun" farming model allows B&W's watercress farms to lie fallow to rest and recharge naturally each year for a smaller ecofootprint and reduced strain on the land and environment. Combined, these seasonal farms qualify the family as the largest watercress growers in the world, though they seem focused more on quality than on size.

Watercress contains a storehouse of nutrients and has been used as a tonic since ancient times to cleanse the blood and liver of toxins and promote an overall feeling of good health. It has been used in a variety of ways, including to enhance stamina, to rid the body of excess fluids, and as a great antioxidant. Hippocrates, the "father of medicine," is said to have established his first hospital close to a watercress stream so that he could use fresh stems to treat his patients. Since that time scientists have identified many of the beneficial compounds contained in the plant.

Watercress is a juicy, vivid green, aquatic plant that is native to Eurasia and was introduced to North America, where it may be found throughout Canada and the United States. The original Latin name of watercress is *Rorippa nasturtium-aquaticum*, which was later changed to *Nasturtium officinale*. Like broccoli, cauliflower, kale, mustard, horseradish, collard greens, turnips, and bok choy, it belongs to the family Cruciferae. For a comprehensive list of the cruciferous vegetables, see chapter 8, "The Forever Young Kitchen."

This hardy perennial is found in abundance near springs, and in open running watercourses, shallow creeks, ditches, ponds, lakes, brooks, and slow-moving rivers—wherever the water is clear and cool and slow-moving. Watercress thrives in shallow (2 to 6 inches), alkaline water in sun or even in pots of rich alluvial soil standing in dishes of water, and it has a creeping habit. The plant has smooth, fleshy stems that bear roundish, heart-shaped leaflets and small white flowers on the extremities. It has been used for thousands of years as a nutritious addition to cuisine and an important factor in herbal medicine. One of the very first plants cultivated by humans, watercress was used by Persian and Greek soldiers as a tonic to improve their health and stamina. Of particular interest to me, the famed seventeenth-century English herbalist Nicholas Culpeper recommended this bitter, pungent, stimulant herb to "free the face" from blotches, spots, and blemishes. In North America, Native Americans used watercress for liver and kidney trouble and to dissolve gallstones.

Watercress has risen to a much-deserved starring role in elaborate culinary preparations. The good news is that it is both beneficial for the health and tasty to the palate. As mentioned, it is a popular garnish, and it is delicious in salads. It is also a delightful addition to herb butters, dressings, casseroles, soups, and sauces for fish, as well as making refreshing and nourishing teas. The ancient Romans enjoyed, as do their descendants, watercress dressed with olive oil and vinegar. Some of the constituents of watercress are volatile oil, flavonoids, phosphorus, nitrogen, beta-carotene, lutein, iodine, protein, folic acid, and sulfur (which probably accounts for the herb's pungent fragrance). It is particularly rich in iron, calcium, potassium, and vitamin C and includes many other valuable mineral and vitamins. For a selection of great watercress recipes, see chapter 8.

Beneficial Uses

Watercress is believed to be an effective diuretic that promotes urine flow, which helps in clearing toxins from the system. The diuretic properties help relieve excess water retention and edema, and it was historically used in heart failure to remove retained fluid. It is also thought to support good kidney function and ease urinary and bladder problems. People of many cultures have also used watercress to break up kidney or bladder stones.

Herbalists have employed watercress to clear toxins from the body.

Watercress is useful in treating skin eruptions, eczema, acne, rashes, and other skin infections.

In addition, watercress is considered a tonic for the liver. The herb has been used to promote bile production and flow, which supports liver function, eases gallbladder complaints, and is also beneficial to the digestive system. The herb has been thought to alleviate indigestion and inhibit gas formation.

In Victorian England, before oranges became affordable, watercress was eaten to ward off scurvy. Indeed, the plant gained the nickname "poor man's bread" in reference to the working-class tradition of starting the day with a watercress sandwich—or just watercress if bread was too expensive! Its high vitamin C content also helps correct other imbalances due to vitamin C deficiency.

Watercress is thought to be an effective expectorant that helps to expel excess mucus and is believed to relieve bronchitis, coughs, and mucus in the lungs.

The high biologically available iron content in watercress is thought to be useful in cases of anemia, and iron, coupled with watercress's high folic acid content, made the herb a staple recommendation for pregnant women in the early 1900s.

Watercress is loaded with nutrients and has been considered an overall tonic for good health. It has been used to ease the debility associated with chronic disease; to increase physical endurance, supporting the ancient soldiers' use of the herb to enhance the body's immune system; and to stimulate the body's metabolism.

Watercress was used in the past to help in cases of tuberculosis, and recent studies have found that it may be effective against cultures of the tubercle bacillus.

The flavonoids in watercress are said to increase immunity, and research shows promise in studying watercress's potential role in cancer prevention and treatment. It is nature's richest source of a specific volatile mustard oil, phenylethyl isothiocyanate (PEITC), shown in many animal, and of late human, studies to fight cancer cells.

Watercress, the New Ancient Superfood

Key research findings on watercress and health and nutrition include:

- Watercress is a cruciferous vegetable, and population studies associate an increased intake of cruciferous vegetables with reduced risk of cancers at several sites, including the breast and prostate.
- Daily consumption of watercress results in a significant decrease in lymphocyte (white blood cell) DNA damage; DNA damage is an important event in cancer development.
- Watercress is a rich source of the glucosinolate derivatives phenethyl isothiocyanate (PEITC) and methylsulphinylakyl isothiocyanates (MEITCs), which have a range of anticancer activities.
- Beneficial effects against the three key stages of carcinogenesis (initiation, proliferation, and metastasis) were observed in a study involving watercress extract and colon cancer cells.
- When smokers ate watercress with each meal for three days, the activation of a key carcinogen in tobacco was inhibited.
- An in vitro study involving breast cancer cells found that the addition of a watercress extract inhibited their invasive potential.
- A study investigating the effects of a diet supplemented with PEITC in mice grafted with human prostate tumors resulted in a 50 percent reduction in tumor weight.
- Watercress is a good source of key nutrients and carotenoids, including lutein and beta-carotene, associated with the maintenance of eye and skin health. Daily consumption of watercress increases plasma lutein levels by 100 percent and beta-carotene levels by 33 percent. Daily watercress consumption has been shown to decrease plasma triglyceride levels by about 10 percent.

- Watercress is rich in vitamin A (via beta-carotene) and vitamin C and a source of folate, calcium, iron, and vitamin E. It also contains a variety of phytochemicals including glucosinolates, lutein, flavonoids, and hydroxycinamic acids. As discussed in chapter 2, the flavor cinnamic aldehyde contains Michael acceptor pharmacophores, which turn on gene expression of a number of cell-protective antioxidant enzymes. Cinnamic aldehyde in both cell culture and animal studies is looking promising as a therapeutic agent for the deadly skin cancer melanoma.
- Watercress has significant antioxidant activity in vitro. Eighty grams of watercress, one cereal bowl full, provides one of the "at least five a day" portions of fruit and vegetables.
- Watercress is recommended by the U.S. Department of Health and Human Services to help reduce the risk of many chronic diseases.
- As a low-calorie vegetable, watercress may play a role in weight management. And 85 percent of watercress's calories are in the form of protein, an extremely high amount.
- Nutrients and phytochemicals in fruit and vegetables appear to work synergistically.

Cancer Protection/Antioxidant

The mix of nutrients and phytochemicals in watercress makes it a valuable food throughout life as part of a healthy diet and lifestyle. I find watercress particularly exciting for its powerful antioxidant and cancer preventing properties. An important study published in *The American Journal of Clinical Nutrition* found that in addition to reducing blood cell DNA damage, a daily serving of watercress increased the ability of blood cells to resist further DNA damage caused by free radicals.

The dietary trial involved thirty healthy men and thirty healthy women (including thirty smokers) eating an 85-gram bag (a cereal bowl full) of fresh watercress every day for eight weeks. The beneficial changes were greatest among the smokers. This may reflect the greater toxic burden or oxidative stress among the smokers, who had significantly lower antioxidant levels at the start of the study than the nonsmokers.

Professor Ian Rowland, who led the research project, said, "Our findings are highly significant. Population studies have shown links between higher intakes of cruciferous vegetables, like watercress, and a reduced risk of a number of cancers, though such studies don't give direct information about causal effects. What makes this study unique is it involves people eating watercress in easily achievable amounts, to see what impact that might have on known biomarkers of cancer risk, such as DNA damage." In other words, you don't need megadoses to get results.

Since the pioneering work by Professor Stephen Hecht in 1995, when he demonstrated that eating watercress neutralized a cancer-causing chemical found in the blood of smokers, there have been many studies linking watercress to potent anticancer activities. Most have been test-tube studies, some have been in animals, and in 2001, there was one in humans, when Professor Rowland showed that eating a bowl of watercress a day significantly reduced DNA damage in blood cells—and DNA damage is thought to be one of the key processes that can lead to the development of cancers. It is DNA damage that triggers cancer cell development, proliferation or uncontrolled growth of cancer cells, and metastasis, the spread of cancer cells. These are the three key stages of carcinogenesis, the process that results in cancer.

How Watercress Prevents Cancer

Recently, two exciting studies were published that provide new insight into the potential anticancer effects of watercress.

These studies were conducted over two years in the United Kingdom, where watercress has long been popular, and link laboratory and clinical research. They were led by Professor Graham Packham at the University of Southampton's School of Medicine at Southampton General Hospital and by Barbara Parry, senior research dietician at the Winchester and Andover Breast Unit at the Royal Hampshire County Hospital.

Professor Packham's main interest was in PEITC (beta-phenethyl isothiocyanate), which gives watercress its peppery taste. In fact, watercress is nature's richest source of this fascinating compound, long associated with anticancer properties.

Hundreds of research publications from around the world show that PEITC can *slow the growth of or even kill* cancer cells in laboratory and animal experiments. The research team set out to learn more about the ways in which PEITC exerts its effect on cancer cells and, most important, whether eating watercress could have a similar effect on cells in the human body. Professor Packham's group showed that PEITC is able to completely block the function of a protein called hypoxia-inducible factor, or HIF. This plays a critical role in cancer development.

Cancer cells are continually developing in our bodies. But thankfully they very rarely grow to form tumors. As cancer cells multiply to form a tiny tumor, smaller than 5 millimeters across, they invariably outgrow their blood supply and run out of oxygen and nutrients. To get past this roadblock, they send out signals that can trick the surrounding normal tissues into angiogenesis, growing new blood vessels. If they are successful in securing a good blood supply, they rapidly multiply to form a growing tumor. HIF is at the heart of this process, because it turns on blood vessel–promoting factors. Since PEITC, which is found in watercress, can block the function of HIF, watercress might control cancer growth by depriving tumors of this new blood supply. Therefore, one way in which watercress might control cancer growth is by depriving developing tumors of this new blood supply.

The research team went on to show that PEITC may turn off this HIF signal by changing the function of a second protein called 4EBP1.

Importantly, this provided a measurable readout indicating that HIF activity and could be used to find out whether eating watercress could affect this pathway critical to cancer tumor growth. Working with Barbara Parry, Graham led a pilot study using a group of volunteers, all female breast cancer survivors keen to help in research into new ways to fight the disease. The women underwent a period of fasting before eating a pack of watercress (the nice bit!) and then gave regular blood samples for up to twenty-four hours. The research team was able to detect significant levels of PEITC in the blood of all the participants following the watercress meal. Most important, the researchers showed that the function of 4EBP1 in the women's blood cells was indeed significantly affected—that is, the watercress meal led to biologically active compounds, most likely PEITC, getting into the bloodstream and inhibiting the ability of cells to trigger blood vessel development—something critical to the development of a tumor.

Professor Packham said, "This work is of significance since we have discovered more about how PEITC can act to interfere with key pathways in cancer cells. It will be important to confirm the clinical findings in a larger group of individuals, but the results of this pilot study do indicate that eating watercress as part of a normal healthy diet might modulate these pathways within cells in the body. This work does not prove that eating watercress would directly decrease the risk of cancer, but it does take an important step toward understanding the potential health benefits of this crop."

Dr. Steve Rothwell of the Watercress Alliance stated, "We are very excited by the outcome of Professor Packham's work. Many laboratory and animal studies point to the cancer fighting properties of PEITC—and thus indirectly to the benefit of eating nature's richest source of this special chemical—watercress."

But this work goes farther, showing a clear link between eating a serving of watercress and the downregulation of a biochemical pathway that's known to be involved in the development of breast cancer. The inference is that regular consumption of watercress could play a role in reducing the risk of this and other cancers. Later in this chapter we will report on another study that demonstrates how the combination of turmeric and watercress can also help to prevent breast cancer.

The Brassica Family: Key to Cancer Prevention

A study published in the *International Journal of Oncology* demonstrated the link between diet and stress-induced cancer.

Researchers examined the possible growth-promoting effects of the stress-associated hormone norepinephrine on immortalized human pancreatic duct epithelial cells. The results indicated that norepinephrine can increase the proliferation of these cells. Norepinephrine also increased interleukin-6 and vascular endothelial growth factor, both believed to promote cancer of pancreatic duct epithelial cells. Simply put, this demonstrates another verifiable link between stress and cancer.

Armed with this discovery, the researchers began to test the dietary antioxidants sulforaphane and resveratrol to see if they could inhibit norepinephrine-mediated increases in cell proliferation. The results indicated that sulforaphane *but not* resveratrol could do so. The researchers believe that sulforaphane's anticancer activity is related to the induction of phase 2 enzymes such as quinine reductase and glutathione S-transferase, and the enhanced transcription of tumor suppressor proteins.

Sulforaphane, discovered by accident in 1995 by a group of scientists researching the anticancer compounds in broccoli, is a phytochemical compound that can be obtained by eating cruciferous vegetables such as arugula, watercress, brussels sprouts, broccoli, broccoli sprouts, cabbage, cauliflower, bok choy, kale, collards, kohlrabi, mustard, turnip, radish, and rutabaga. Sulforaphane is particularly abundant in watercress and broccoli sprouts.

We know that stress accelerates aging and disease. When you are under stress, your immune system is also compromised, weakening your ability to ward off invading organisms. Chronic stress raises the level of the excitatory hormones, including norepinephrine and cortisol, which can wear your body down and lead to disease. Sulforaphane inhibits the norepinephrine-mediated increase in the interleukin-6 levels in the cells, which is a very good thing. Interleukin-6 is responsible for the shift from acute inflammation to chronic inflammation, the root of so many diseases. Finding a safe and effective substance that can inhibit the overproduction of norepinephrine is a significant accomplishment.

Watercress, Turmeric, and Breast Cancer

Numerous studies validating the cancer-fighting properties of watercress continue to appear in medical journals. Studies include human trials in Germany and the University of Minnesota that indicated that watercress consumption can repair damaged DNA. Studies in the United Kingdom of breast cancer survivors, published in early 2010, have recorded equally impressive results.

Rutgers researchers tested turmeric, and its active ingredient, curcumin (see page 43 for more on this Indian spice), along with phenethyl isothiocyanate (PEITC), a naturally occurring substance particularly abundant in the cruciferous vegetables, especially watercress, cabbage, winter cress, broccoli, brussels sprouts, kale, cauliflower, kohlrabi, and turnips. The discovery was announced in the journal *Cancer Research*. According to Ah-Ng Tony Kong, a professor of pharmaceutics at Rutgers: "The bottom line is that PEITC and curcumin, alone or in combination, demonstrate significant cancer-preventive qualities in laboratory mice, and the combination of PEITC and curcumin could be effective in treating established prostate cancers."

Chocolate: "Gift from the Gods"

The source of all cocoa powder and chocolate is cacao beans, which are found in the pods of the cacao tree, *Theobroma cacao,* an evergreen typically grown within 20 degrees of the equator. To make cocoa and chocolate, the beans are fermented, roasted, shelled, ground, and often combined with a sweetener or flavoring agent.

The cacao tree was originally found in the tropical rain forests of Central America. It was cultivated thousands of years ago by the ancient Aztecs, who believed that the plant was a gift from their gods. In fact, its very name, *Theobroma,* means "of the gods." The tree can grow to forty feet in height and has a very unusual appearance because the football-shaped pods that contain the beans grow directly out of the trunk. So valuable was the fruit of this tree that the Aztecs were using cocoa beans as a form of currency when the Spanish first arrived on the continent.

When Europeans were introduced to this remarkably delicious substance, they were very impressed by the stimulating effects of cocoa extracts and the feelings of well-being they generated. As mentioned earlier in this chapter, cocoa is an excellent source of phytonutrients known as catechins and, like tea and blueberries, controls gene expression by turning off damaging transcription factors such as NF-κB and turning on protective transcription factors such as NRF2.

Phytonutrient-rich chocolate and the cocoa it is made from are complex foods containing more than three hundred compounds and chemicals in each bite. These exert powerful effects on brain chemistry, specifically serotonin, dopamine, and opiate peptides, resulting in a positive mood and euphoric feelings. Chocolate stimulates the release of brain opiates known as endorphins, which are chemically similar to morphine; in fact, the brain responds to them in the same way as it responds to morphine. These brain opiates are largely responsible for the body's response to pleasure, stress, and pain.

Love at First Bite

It is now believed that cravings for sweet and high-fat foods like chocolate may be partly mediated by these brain opiates. One substance in chocolate, phenylethylamine, mimics the action of these natural opiates and gives us the feeling of being in love. Perhaps that is why chocolate is the gift associated with Valentine's Day. We may indulge in chocolate after a failed relationship and a broken heart to reproduce that incomparable feeling. The natural antidepressant effect of chocolate is one of the many benefits we receive when enjoying a piece of dark chocolate. Chocolate is also rich in oleic acid, the monounsaturated fat found in olive oil, which helps us absorb important nutrients.

For optimum health benefits and enjoyment, choose extra-dark chocolate—at least 70% to 85% cocoa content. Also choose non-Dutched cocoa, as the process of alkalinization or "Dutching" cocoa significantly reduces the amount of flavonols in cocoa. By weight, cocoa has more antioxidants than blueberries, green tea, or red wine. Chocolate and cocoa protect the cardiovascular system, significantly reducing the incidence of atherosclerosis. Chocolate is also similar to the blueberry in that it affords protection to our brain. As we know, substances that are neuroprotective are also therapeutic to the skin.

Skin Science and Cocoa

When ingested orally, cocoa has potent neuroprotective effects, the result of specific micronutrients. The neuroprotective effects of cocoa are derived from the cocoa procyanidin fraction, which is extracted from cocoa powder using natural solvents that then become rich in these active molecules. The solvents, now rich in the flavonoids and procyanidins, display powerful activity in the cell and affect gene expression in a very positive way.

Scientists have found that procyanidin B-2 protects brain cells from inflammation and are looking at the cocoa procyanidin fraction and procyanidin B-2 to prevent and treat Alzheimer's disease.

My interest in the cocoa procyanidin fractions, and specifically pro-cyanidin B-2, lies in their protective effects and therapeutic efficacy when applied to skin. The skin is our interface between our bodies and the world. Unfortunately, it is under constant bombardment by external stressors, including the environment, UV and electromagnetic radia-tion, air pollution, and chemical irritants, as well as internal stressors, including poor diet, alcohol ingestion, smoking, and stress, to name a few. Procyanidin B-2 is a powerful anti-inflammatory that can switch off the production of the pro-inflammatory chemicals that are released in the skin by these stressors.

The Birth of a Wrinkle

Excess exposure to ultraviolet radiation is hugely damaging to the skin. It increases free-radical activity in the cell plasma membrane, which releases arachidonic acid, the precursor of numerous pro-inflammatory chemicals including the prostaglandins and HETEs. This activates transcription factors such as NF-κB and AP-1. These in turn upregulate negative genes that produce pro-inflammatory cytokines that damage skin cells. When transcription factors such as AP-1 are activated, they produce and release collagen-digesting proteins (matrix metalloprotein-ase), resulting in microscarring in the deep portion of the skin called the dermis. The multiple *micro*-scars lead to *macro*-scarring, and this is "the birth of a wrinkle."

The Death of a Wrinkle

The cocoa procyanidin fractions, including procyanidin B-2, upset the wrinkle-producing process. They prevent the oxidation of lipids in the cell plasma membrane, blocking the production of arachidonic acid, while at the same time inhibiting the activation of the transcription

THE EXTREME NO-SUN-EXPOSURE PRESCRIPTION

For years I have recommended that people have no unprotected sun exposure, as have all of my colleagues in dermatology. This recommendation was made because of the pro-inflammatory, photo-aging, and cancer-causing effects of ultraviolet light. If the skin is the only organ we are concerned with, this is good advice, but dermatologists, like other subspecialists, can often fail to see the implications of treating a single organ system at the expense of other vital organs.

We now know that vitamin D, the sunshine vitamin, is produced by sunlight on the skin. It is then absorbed and circulated in the bloodstream. Vitamin D is stored mainly in the liver and must be processed by the liver and kidneys before it is converted to the active form.

Vitamin D is also present in cold-water fish, another good reason to consume that delicious piece of salmon. Dietary sources of vitamin D are often inadequate to meet our minimum needs, and this is now resulting in an epidemic of subchronic vitamin D deficiency diseases.

Vitamin D is known to enhance all vital organs and reduce the risk of all forms of cancer throughout the body. Scientists now recognize that low vitamin D levels increase the risk of cardiovascular disease and mental depression, as well as the obvious disease, osteoporosis. Laboratory tests are revealing very low levels of vitamin D in adults, increasing our risk for multiple age-related diseases. Supplementation with vitamin D capsules is an unexplored area, and I believe will prove to be nowhere near as effective or safe as getting vitamin D from sun exposure. I advise my patients to get moderate amounts of sun exposure, unprotected by clothing or sunscreens, on a regular basis. This does not mean sitting in the sun until the skin shows signs of redness. We can slowly increase our exposure as the protective melanin in the skin increases with repeated exposure. Each person is different, so use caution and don't overdo it. The goal is not to get a suntan or bake in the sun.

For sunbathing to be effective, our skin must contain adequate natural oils. I recommend not showering or bathing before taking a therapeutic sunbath. After sunbathing, these oils need to be absorbed into the skin and to enter the tiny blood vessels called the dermal vasculature, so the deal is not to shower for at least eight hours after sun exposure. By following this technique, we can produce thousands of units of vitamin D that the body can utilize, without the fear of overdose seen with oral supplementation.

---

factors NF-κB and AP-1. These remarkable procyanidins also prevent apoptosis.

Spin Traps

Spin traps are molecules that have been used as research tools to study free radicals. Since free radicals exist for only a fraction of a second, it is very difficult to study these reactive molecules, whether in the test tube or the human body. However, when free radicals are caught in a spin trap, scientists are able to study and measure them. Spin traps are proving to be very helpful in preventing and treating disease.

When free radicals are captured by spin traps, they become inactivated, unable to do their normal damage. This means that they are prevented from damaging the delicate portion of the cell known as the cell plasma membrane. One type of spin trap currently under study is phenyl-butyl-nitrone (PBN), which hails from a group of spin traps known as nitrones. Two scientists, Dr. John Carney of the University of Kentucky and Dr. Robert Floyd of the Oklahoma Research Foundation, have worked with nitrones to treat stroke patients. During a stroke, the brain is deprived of oxygen (ischemia); when blood flow and oxygen resume, a tremendous burst of free-radical activity is generated. The cell plasma membrane area of the nerve cells becomes damaged, resulting in an intense inflammatory response. When the scientists administered nitrone spin traps to stroke patients, they noticed a significant decrease in the incidence of such problems as paralysis and loss of speech.

Dr. Floyd has continued to work with derivatives of PBN and has discovered that these agents also have anticancer activity. It appears that the nitrone spin traps are efficacious in preventing precancers and cancers in the liver of animal models. Derivatives of PBN also appear to be effective against colon cancer and certain forms of brain cancer. Additionally, he has had success in preventing hearing loss resulting from exposure to loud noise, known as acute acoustical trauma.

One of the persistent themes in Dr. Floyd's journal articles is the unknown mechanism of action of the nitrone spin traps. Spin traps exhibit moderate antioxidant activity, but Dr. Floyd does not believe that the antioxidant effects are the sole reason for their anticancer benefits or their protective actions observed in other disease models. Though he admits that he doesn't know their precise mechanism of action and why PBNs possess anticancer activity, he does attest that their positive effects are genuine.

In looking at the molecular structure of the PBN nitrone spin traps, I recognized a familiar structure, one that is seen in the Michael acceptor pharmacophores in cinnamic aldehyde, the curcuminoids found in turmeric, and the nitroalkenes described earlier in this chapter.

As for cinnamic aldehyde, the curcuminoids, and the nitroalkenes, I believe the anticancer activity and other therapeutic benefits of a nitrone spin trap results from the fact that it is a mild electrophile and a Michael acceptor pharmacophore. As we know, strong electrophiles are damaging. But mild electrophiles can actually work to our benefit, as they activate NRF2 while inhibiting the activation of the pro-inflammatory transcription factor NF-κB. The net result is the suppression of the production of the pro-inflammatory cytokines and the supraphysiological release of nitric oxide, which can lead to tumor formation and progression.

The therapeutic benefits of PBN derive not simply from antioxidant action but from the activation of gene expression, just as those of the phytonutrients do. When I presented this nitrone spin trap mechanism of action hypothesis to Dr. Floyd, he wasn't quite convinced, but I believe that he and his colleagues are seriously considering this explanation.

You have learned about the mechanisms by which a number of superstar nutrients not only promote positive gene expression but also protect you from damage and disease. These nutrients will appear again in the following chapter, "The Metabolic Miracle."

The next chapter will offer you a simple plan—a metabolic miracle you can perform to lose unwanted body fat safely, quickly, and permanently. You will learn about the importance of retaining muscle mass as you lose weight and age, the relationship between sleep deprivation and weight gain, and a new nutritional power food to add to your diet. Aside from helping you lose health-threatening visceral fat, the metabolic miracle plan will leave you energized, optimistic, and luminous.

Chapter Three

THE METABOLIC MIRACLE:
LOSING FAT, PRESERVING MUSCLE AND BONE

With obesity on the rise in America, weight loss has become a national obsession. We are awash in a plethora of different weight-loss programs and countless weight-loss supplements. Unfortunately, rather than waning, obesity appears to be on the rise, so it is no surprise that we are a nation obsessed with dieting, diet books, diet foods, and diet fads. Our quest for weight loss is as unending as it is unsuccessful.

But who knew that that hard-earned 5-, 10-, or more-pound weight loss was destroying both muscle and bone, with far-reaching deleterious effects? The fact is that the wrong kind of dieting increases our levels of inflammatory markers and accelerates the loss of precious muscle mass. Unfortunately, this is not the only problem with conventional dieting/weight loss "wisdom." Dieting is a key culprit in declining bone mass density (BMD). We are never informed that weight loss, including loss facilitated surgically through gastric bypass or banding procedures, has been repeatedly documented as depleting bone density and increasing fracture risk.

Risky Business

I was a coinvestigator on a study on sarcopenia, the progressive loss of muscle tissue with age, titled "Sarcopenia: When Weight Loss Is Counter-Productive" with colleagues including Harry Preuss, M.D. M.A.C.N., C.N.S., at the Department of Physiology, Georgetown University Medical Center. The idea that weight loss in an otherwise healthy person could be counterproductive seems hard to believe, but as you will discover, the wrong kind of weight loss can wreak havoc on both your muscle tissue and your bones.

Skeletal muscle mass and strength generally peak between 20 and 35 years of age. From then on, 3 to 8 percent of muscle mass may be lost per decade, a loss rate that has previously been reported to accelerate after the age of 60. We have long known that with each passing decade we tend to lose 5 pounds of muscle mass and gain 10 pounds of body fat. My own research has shown that dieting can speed up this loss.

As we age, we develop an increased risk for osteopenia and osteoporosis. Osteopenia can be defined as the thinning of bone mass, most common in postmenopausal women due to a lack of estrogen. This decrease in bone mass is not usually considered severe, but it is considered a very serious risk factor for the development of osteoporosis. Health experts are well aware that osteopenia and osteoporosis are consequences of the age-related decline in bone density, but few are cognizant of the deleterious effects of sarcopenia.

In this chapter, I will tell you about a "metabolic miracle," an efficient way to say good-bye to body fat. In these pages you will learn the secret of body fat, how to minimize the risks of weight loss, and how to prevent and/or reverse this trend of muscle and bone density loss. You will gain a new understanding of the role that toxins play in weight gain and how to beat them at their own game.

Understanding Sarcopenia and the Importance of Muscle Versus Fat

Sarcopenia differs from the involuntary muscle depletion that is seen when our nutrition is inadequate or caused by starvation or diseases like cancer or AIDS. It is also distinct from cachexia, a cytokine-driven loss of lean body mass that occurs despite maintenance of body weight. Sarcopenia is sometimes seen in patients with rheumatoid arthritis, congestive heart failure, or renal (kidney) failure. As Ronenn Roubenoff and Carmen Castaneda wrote in a paper titled "Sarcopenia—Understanding the Dynamics of Aging Muscle," published in *The Journal of the American Medical Association,* "Sarcopenia is not a disease . . . but is the backdrop against which the drama of disease is played out: a body already depleted of protein because of aging is less able to withstand the protein catabolism that comes with acute illness or inadequate protein intake." As you will learn in the Metabolic Miracle diet described in these pages, supplying protein in an efficient absorbable form with the right supportive nutrients can sustain muscle and reverse the trend of catabolism, or breakdown.

Although cachexia generally connotes a state of advanced malnutrition and wasting, we now know that this term refers more specifically to a loss of body cell mass. Studies of starvation, critical illness, and normal aging have found that a loss of body cell mass greater than 40 percent is fatal. Even with as little as 5 percent loss of body cell mass, there are demonstrable changes in morbidity (a diseased state), including loss of muscle strength, altered energy metabolism, and increased susceptibility to infections. Accompanying the muscle loss is a reduction in voluntary strength, about 30 percent between 50 and 70 years of age.

With the huge number of baby boomers aged 50-plus, we know how important it is to prevent this loss of critical muscle mass. Fortunately, this generation has a penchant for physical fitness. As I often write, we don't have to age like our parents. We have a choice, and my great joy in writing *Forever Young* is letting readers know their options. **Too often we think of flabby, sagging muscles, potbellies, and excess body fat as simply an aesthetic problem. Nothing could be further from the truth. Body fat is toxic, and the loss of precious muscle mass and bone is equally deleterious to health and well-being.**

The word "sarcopenia" is derived from the Greek root words *sarx*, meaning "flesh," and *penia*, meaning "loss." Sarcopenia has important consequences for balance, metabolism, physical appearance, general well-being, and quality of life. As the length of the human life span increases, the number of people suffering from sarcopenia is also projected to increase. Sarcopenia causes many problems because as it progresses, our mobility is further impaired, impeding the normal activities of daily living. This can result in osteoporosis, falls, fractures, thrombophlebitis, pulmonary embolism, isolation, depression, and other adverse consequences. An estimated 14 percent of people between the ages of 65 and 75 require assistance with the normal activities of daily living, and this figure increases to 45 percent for persons over 85 years of age. The medical effects and economic costs of sarcopenia are profound, and, as one reviewer has reported, "Sarcopenia is an important cause of frailty, disability, and loss of independence in the elderly, and recent estimates suggest that it costs the United States over $18 billion per year, a sum on par with the economic consequences of osteoporosis."

A Deadly Duo

Some studies suggest that sarcopenia is the major predictor of function limitations, while others suggest that it is the combination of obesity and sarcopenia that is the primary cause of disability. The implications are that the dangerous combination of sarcopenia and obesity in old age is more strongly associated with disability in daily living than either sarcopenia or obesity alone. As you can see, the implications for disaster are enormous and the quality of life is severely compromised when muscle mass has been replaced with toxic body fat. The goal of the Perricone Forever Young Program is to keep you strong, fit, and active while maintaining a healthy weight.

Healthy Weight—
Pulling the Scales from Our Eyes

Most people assume a healthy weight can be determined by the reading on the bathroom scale. But this is not an accurate assessment. It is not the *amount* of weight you lose that is the most important measure of well-being but rather the *kind* of weight you lose. The secret in determining healthy weight is your body composition index (BCI). If you gain 2 pounds of lean muscle mass and lose 2 pounds of body fat, your scale weight will not have changed, but you will be in better shape. Your goal is to lose body fat and maintain and/or restore muscle mass—not the other way around.

For overall beneficial health, health professionals and scientists do not pretend to know how many pounds of muscle it takes to offset gains in body fat or how much fat one has to lose to offset losses in muscle. What is clear is that loss of lean muscle and gain of body fat are clearly negative treatment outcomes, regardless of any changes in scale weight. **The litmus test of a safe and efficacious weight loss program is the preservation of lean muscle and the depletion of excess body fat—in short, *the kind, not amount*, of weight that is lost.**

The bad news is that some level of sarcopenia exists in *all* older individuals. In the face of acute or chronic illness, maximizing muscle mass and protein stores with adequate nutritional support, as you will learn in the Metabolic Miracle diet that follows, aggressive physical therapy, and exercise programs become all the more important if muscle function and quality of life are to be preserved as we age.

Living in Fat City

What is behind the increasing rate of obesity/sarcopenia plaguing the world? There are many reasons for it, foremost among them the superabundance of junk and processed "food" available today, so let us consider a few possibilities.

The primary treatment for improving the muscle/fat ratio is exercise and diet. In the case of muscle, it is generally accepted that most people get too little exercise. No one would disagree that such a state leads to a smaller muscle mass and a larger fat mass. As for the fat factor, dietary indiscretion is rampant everywhere. The public was first trained to focus on the saturated fat content of foods to avoid atherosclerosis and heart disease. Never mind that trans fats were ignored; excess calories and refined carbohydrates that often replaced the avoided saturated fats were also ignored. Consuming refined sugar, white flour, and other simple carbohydrates causes your insulin level to spike, because these carbohydrates break down quickly and turn into glucose in your bloodstream. Insulin regulates fat storage. When insulin levels are elevated, we store fat in adipose tissue; when they are low, fat is used as fuel. What you eat helps to maintain the right hormonal balance to produce energy at a steady level. Complex carbohydrates like whole grains, fresh fruits, vegetables, and beans are digested more slowly, leading to gradual and smaller increases in insulin. What you eat is used as energy for your body rather than stored as fat.

I have always contended that pro-inflammatory, easily digestible (high-glycemic) simple carbohydrates, not dietary fat, saturated or otherwise, are the major cause of obesity, heart disease, and many other chronic diseases of civilization, perhaps even sarcopenia. The message of reducing calories and avoiding fat has gained so much popularity that it is possible that such a diet may lead to even more sarcopenia. The unfortunate surfeit of nonfat and low-fat diets has been responsible for widespread avoidance of good fats like the omega-3s, which can be a factor in today's widespread depression and obesity, because we need healthy fats to metabolize fat.

In my first book, *The Wrinkle Cure,* and the seven that followed, I described a diet high in pro-inflammatory, high-glycemic foods— refined sugars and starches—as the culprit and causative factor in elevated blood sugar and insulin levels and resulting inflammation. This chronic, low-grade, subclinical inflammation is at the root of obesity and a host of age-related diseases and degenerative conditions from bone loss to sarcopenia, from arthritis to Alzheimer's, and so forth.

Getting Off the Roller-Coaster Ride

When we are overweight or obese, there is a constant exchange of fat for muscle. Improper dieting will greatly accelerate this exchange, because we have reduced our overall caloric intake. When we are significantly overweight, we experience chronically high insulin levels, which start to drop as soon as we start to diet. Though this might sound like a good thing, it is, in fact somewhat of a catch-22. Though low levels of insulin will decrease inflammation, allowing us to utilize the body fat for energy, insulin is required to bring protein into the cells to maintain muscle mass, a process known as the anabolic effect. Since overweight people have chronically high levels of circulating insulin, they become insensitive to decreased levels and cannot recognize these new lower levels. In this state, their bodies are unable to trigger the amino acid uptake needed to maintain muscle mass. Insulin is needed to take up both glucose and amino acids into the muscle. In addition to the loss of critical muscle and bone, being overweight or obese also increases your risk for type 2 diabetes. When we have excess body fat, we also have higher levels of inflammatory markers such as C-reactive protein and some of the interleukins. Transcription factors like NF-κB are also activated. Once NF-κB is activated, we become insulin-resistant.

This is why it is essential to take a powerful anti-inflammatory approach to dieting. Inflammatory chemicals like NF-κB block the effects of insulin—whether metabolizing blood sugar or nourishing muscles with amino acids. As I said before, the inflammation must be treated first. It is important to note that overexercising can further put us into a catabolic state, in which complex molecules are broken down into simpler ones. This happens because active muscles require more nutrients.

Easy as NBC

When we follow an anti-inflammatory diet, we begin to affect the glucose/insulin system in a positive way. Proper insulin metabolism, in contrast to insulin resistance, favors fat loss and muscle gain. Fortunately, many safe, natural substances can favorably influence the glucose insulin system. I performed a study with Dr. Harry Preuss and colleagues using trivalent chromium in the form of niacin-bound chromium (NBC). Niacin-bound chromium is a substance known to overcome peripheral insulin resistance. Twenty overweight African-American women participated in a randomized, double-blind, placebo-controlled, crossover study. They received a placebo three times a day during the control period and niacin-bound chromium, 200 micrograms three times a day, during the test period for two months. Body weight and fat and nonfat body mass were estimated. Body-weight losses were essentially the same in both the placebo and chromium-receiving subjects, but fat loss was significantly *greater* and nonfat body mass loss significantly *less* with chromium intake. Niacin-bound chromium given to modestly dieting and exercising African-American women caused a significant loss of fat and sparing of muscle compared with those on the placebo, even though the scale-weight losses were essentially similar. A frequent complaint during the study was the lack of a significant decrease in scale weight, but often, in the same breath, the subject would mention a decrease in dress size! That is because muscle is leaner and denser than fat, and the subjects were losing fat.

At this point, let us focus more on maintaining muscle mass. With typical everyday movement and exercise, skeletal muscle in the human body is under constant renovation. An equal balance between synthesis and degradation of muscle proteins results in the size of muscle tissue remaining essentially unchanged. If there is a shift in this balance, the resulting state will be atrophy, when breakdown is greater than synthesis, or hypertrophy, when synthesis is greater than breakdown. It follows that changes in muscle mass are correlated with modifications in protein synthesis, protein degradation, or both. During and immediately following exercise, degradation of muscle protein is increased. The released amino acids that result from protein breakdown have the potential to produce ATP, a nucleotide derived from adenosine that is present in muscle tissue and is the major source of energy for cellular reactions. This means that there is less protein when the stressed muscles come to rest. After vigorous exercise, especially weight-bearing, cells go through a 30- to 60-minute window in which amino acid uptake can increase, dramatically building muscle. By ingesting high-quality, readily absorbable (high-protein efficiency rating, or PER) protein, we can gain the most muscle-building benefits; if we miss that window, our amino acid uptake goes back to the baseline and the benefits of protein ingestion drop tremendously.

In addition, damage to some muscle cell membranes may occur, creating delayed-onset muscle soreness. This is especially associated with eccentric exercise such as downhill running. Injury can occur in the connective tissue as well, diminishing performance for some time. Obviously, lessening the protein breakdown will ameliorate this situation, at least to some extent. Shortening the period of increased protein degradation is advantageous for people wishing to maintain and even improve their muscle mass. The fact that sarcopenia is a multifactorial

CLOCK WORK—
THE KEY TO BEAUTIFUL SKIN AND HEALTHY WEIGHT

I have often written about the importance of sleep for health and beauty, including numerous blogs on the Huffington Post. Providing a wonderful service to readers of her blog, Arianna Huffington has been very vocal about the importance of sleep. Right after New Year's, Arianna posted a Sleep Challenge 2010 to raise awareness about the serious problem of women suffering from sleep deprivation. Now more than ever, women have tremendous demands on their time and, as a consequence, suffer greatly from the lack of sleep. As you will discover, insufficient sleep seriously disrupts our health, our weight, our sense of well-being, and our skin.

Sleeping Beauties

As some of the world's most beautiful and talented actresses converged on the red carpet at the 2010 Oscars, many wondered how they did it, looking so radiant and wonderful despite the grueling schedules they keep. This year's nominees included Helen Mirren, Sandra Bullock, Meryl Streep, Penélope Cruz, Mo'Nique, Carey Mulligan, Maggie Gyllenhaal, Gabourey Sidibe, Vera Farmiga, and Anna Kendrick, whose ages ranged from the early twenties to the early sixties, proving once again how ageless beauty can be.

Regardless of age, each star has her own unique style. And though I cannot profess to know their secrets, I can share with you some of my own secrets for radiant skin and a healthy body weight—it all starts with our internal clock and a good night's sleep.

We humans are creatures of habit, for better or worse. We like to eat our meals at the same time, go to bed at the same time, and so on. There is an excellent reason for this. We all need to follow a daily circadian rhythm—that is, a rhythm based on the twenty-four-hour cycle, the time it takes the earth to make a full rotation on its axis.

For thousands of years this was not a problem: humans went to sleep when the sun went down and arose when the sun came up. But those days are long gone. It has become apparent that this is not a positive change, as scientists have discovered that disruption of this cycle causes us to develop a number of metabolic discords.

Staying up too late, snacking throughout the day, and skipping meals all upset the genes that control daily rhythms in the brain and throughout the body. One important finding is that the "clock," which scientists thought was only in the central part of the brain, is also present in the part of the brain that controls appetite. In fact, biological clocks function not only in the brain but in many other parts of the body as well. They govern not only the sleep cycle but also functions including fluid balance, body temperature, oxygen consumption—and now, it has been shown, appetite. Researchers at Northwestern University and the Howard Hughes Medical Institute have identified wide-ranging molecular and behavioral changes in mice that have a faulty circadian system. In people, similar changes in body fat and metabolic activity are known as metabolic syndrome.

Fred W. Turek, a member of the research team, stated that the study provided new genetic evidence that physiological outputs of the biological clock, sleep, and appetite are interconnected at the molecular and behavioral levels.

This research data give new credence to the concept that we are creatures of habit. Perhaps more important, it establishes the fact that we need to follow a regimen in our daily lives, one based on cycles as primary as the rising and setting of the sun, to which humans have been acclimated since the dawn of civilization. Though it is not practical to go to bed with the sun, it does make sense to get up with it, and this provides us with a good excuse not to stay up to all hours and become sleep-deprived. Not getting sufficient high-quality sleep has been linked to increased appetite and unwanted weight gain.

Sleep to Lose Weight

An important study at the University of Chicago demonstrated that sleep deprivation causes us to overeat, because it disrupts the balance between two appetite-related hormones—ghrelin and leptin. When we don't get enough sleep, our levels of ghrelin, a hormone produced by stomach cells and believed to increase feelings of hunger, rise. Leptin, a hormone produced by our fat cells that suppresses appetite and burns fat stores, is decreased.

Even worse, the most sleep-deprived people in the study craved fattening, carbohydrate-rich foods, such as cookies, cake, candy, pasta, and muffins. According to Dr. Eve Van Cauter, the lead researcher, these cravings are the result of elevated levels of the stress hormone cortisol. When we are fully rested, our cortisol levels drop; sleep deprivation has the unfortunate opposite effect. The study participants also metabolized glucose less efficiently. Dr. Van Cauter reported that the effects of sleep deprivation on glucose metabolism are similar to those found in the elderly. She therefore concluded that chronic sleep deprivation may have long-term harmful effects on the body—not the least of which are weight gain and possibly accelerated aging as well.

As with exercising, we need to establish regular, healthy habits and regimens. We should strive to get close to eight hours of sleep per night and learn not to skip meals, including breakfast. Implementing these simple rules will eliminate the pro-inflammatory habits we tend to fall into and help us achieve and maintain optimum weight.

condition may explain why it can be treated by several different means other than resistance training. These include hormonal interventions, increased high-PER protein in the diet, and nutritional supplements.

Some Hormones Are Not a Good Option

The most accepted hormonal treatment for sarcopenia is growth hormone (GH). Patients with sarcopenia have been found to have reduced levels of growth hormones. One study in which patients with sarcopenia were treated with GH supplements showed a significant increase in plasma IGF-1 levels and small increases in lean body mass. Unfortunately, serious side effects followed, including increased levels of circulating glucose and higher systolic blood pressure. Other adverse side effects included carpal tunnel syndrome; gynecomastia, or excessive development of the breasts in males; and hyperglycemia. Although GH therapy significantly increases lean muscle mass, its cons are far greater than its pros. The frequent occurrences of serious side effects as well as the high monetary costs outweigh the clinical benefits. A potential option to replace GH therapy is the use of growth hormone–releasing hormone (GHRH) supplements. GHRH appears to produce the benefits of GH with fewer side effects than with GH therapy.

Testosterone and estrogen supplements are another form of hormonal intervention for elderly people with sarcopenia. One study showed that testosterone replacement therapy increased grip strength and decreased low-density lipoprotein cholesterol with no detectable changes in weight, body fat, or lean muscle mass. Unfortunately, the results show too much variability for testosterone therapy to be recommended confidently for sarcopenia. Like testosterone, estrogen or estradiol replacement therapy also yields variable results that require further elucidation. The variability may be due to biological differences among people.

Along similar lines, dehydroepiandrosterone (DHEA), an adrenal androgen that is the biological precursor of active androgenic hormones like testosterone and dihydrotestosterone, has been used as replacement therapy to increase the anabolic hormones that augment lean muscle mass in elderly people with sarcopenia. Although widely available as a supplement, DHEA supplementation requires more information and testing before its therapeutic benefits can be ascertained definitively. To sum up, hormone replacement therapy appears to have nominal and variable effects on lean muscle mass and muscle strength, with frequent unfavorable side effects.

Branched-Chain Amino Acids

Another strategy for building lean muscle mass, over and above increasing high-protein-efficiency-rated protein intake, is supplementing with the branch-chain amino acids. The branch-chain amino acids valine, leucine, and isoleucine have been administered to test subjects with positive results. For many years, scientists have been impressed with the ability of leucine, valine, and isoleucine to augment muscle mass. These amino acids yield anabolic effects similar in many respects to those of insulin. Leucine seems to be the most important of the three in building muscle. Leucine is not synthesized by the human body and must be acquired through diet, placing it in the category of an essential amino acid.

In working with young athletes, a balanced intake of all three of these amino acids, along with omega-3 supplements, gave excellent results and kept them away from illegal and dangerous anabolic steroids. I recommend taking the branched-chain amino acids, which are widely available in capsule form, to protect muscle mass.

Chia Seeds:
Omega-3 Fatty Acids and Nutritional Power Food

No discussion of weight loss would be complete without the omega-3 essential fatty acids. Your body needs the right fats to burn fats rather then store them. As you learned in chapter 2, the omega-3s activate nuclear receptors called peroxisome proliferator-activated receptors, or PPARs. These receptors, located in the cell nucleus, control blood sugar, the storing and burning of body fat, and the way energy is used in the body. The omega-3s produce a protein known as *uncoupling protein 3*, which uncouples oxidative phosphorylation. This results in greater energy dissipation as heat and a decrease in stored body fat.

Traditionally, I have recommended consuming foods rich in the omega-3s, such as wild salmon, sardines, anchovies, and so on, as well as taking high-quality fish oil capsules. I cannot repeat often enough that the omega-3s are vital to the health of many organ systems, including the skin, heart, and brain. They are also indispensable in any successful weight loss program.

I can recommend an outstanding new source of the omega-3s: chia seeds. I call them "new" only because they are new to the majority of us, but chia has been used for centuries. I have been working with the Green Foods Corporation to introduce these remarkable seeds, which, as you will soon discover, are unsurpassed for increasing energy, endurance, and much more.

The seeds of the chia plant (*Salvia hispanica L.*) are a concentrated source of high-quality macronutrients required by the body: omega-3 fatty acids, dietary fiber, high-quality complete protein without gluten, and low-glycemic carbohydrates. This outstanding combination of nutrients ensures that I enjoy at least one serving of chia seeds daily.

I suggest that you sprinkle chia seeds on salad, veggies, fruits, cottage cheese, yogurt, main dishes—wherever you can—to take advantage of their tremendous health benefits. They are basically without taste and add crunch when used in this way. They absorb fluid, so if you mix chia seeds in water, they will form a gel, which will add body to salad dressings, sauces, and cooked dishes.

Though micronutrients support all biochemical processes in the body, they are more involved in the structural components of cells and tissues. For example, omega-3 fatty acids are vital components of cellular membranes, while amino acids from protein are needed as integral structural components of muscle tissue, connective tissue, and enzymes, among other functions.

Chia seeds contain micronutrients including substantial amounts of vitamin E and other antioxidants that offer twofold protection, protecting our body and its natural oils from oxidation. Chia seeds are also a good source of bone-building minerals, including calcium, magnesium, and phosphorus, and contain a high level of lignans, phytochemical compounds that act as phytoestrogens. Lignans also possess anticancer properties.

Not only are chia seeds nutritious, they are nonallergenic, contain very little sodium, are gluten-free, and, unlike flax seeds, have been granted GRAS (generally recognized as safe) status by the FDA. Since they possess so many healthful qualities without any known drawbacks, they are gaining well-deserved popularity as a superfood.

Although chia seeds are relatively new to the world food market, they have been a staple food for the peoples of Mexico for centuries. Chia seeds form a hydrophilic colloidal suspension (gel) in water because of their high soluble fiber content. They slowly release their nutrient content and water into the digestive tract for absorption and utilization over extended periods. This provides an even and sustained source of nutrition, hydration, and energy for the body as the gel passes through the digestive tract. Chia seeds were highly valued as an endurance food because of this attribute by the Mayans and Aztecs and are still used today as food in Mexico and the southwestern United States. The ability of chia seeds to form a hydrophilic gel helps in maintaining normal blood sugar levels and promoting gentle detoxification by physically cleaning the lining of the digestive tract during transit.

The Ideal Ratio of Omega Fatty Acids

Chia seeds are an excellent source of both of the essential fatty acids (EFAs), linoleic acid (LA), and the omega-3 fatty acid alpha-linolenic acid (ALA). In fact, chia seeds provide the highest amounts of vegetarian omega-3 fatty acids. They have an ideal omega-6-to-omega-3 ratio of 1:3. Though all omega fatty acids, including omega-3, -6, and -9, contribute to our health, our modern dietary habits often result in many people consuming diets with both an unbalanced ratio of EFAs and not enough omega-3 fatty acids. There are many fatty-acid chemical structures but only two kinds of essential fatty acids: omega-3 and omega-6. Both the absolute and the relative amounts of these fatty acids consumed per day are important, since omega-6 fatty acids may interfere with some of the actions of omega-3 fatty acids, including their anti-inflammatory benefits.

Omega-3 Benefits

Both EPA (eicosapentaenoic acid) and DHA (docosahexaenoic acid) omega-3 fatty acids are essential to our health. DHA is the most abundant fatty acid in the brain and retina, and low levels of it are associated with a decline in learning and memory (which are reversed by the addition of DHA to the diet), age-related cognitive decline, and Alzheimer's disease. In addition, DHA's ability to lower blood fats, known as triglycerides, helps protect against heart disease. Since cardiovascular function and blood flow are often impaired in people with senile dementia, DHA may help improve age-related cognitive decline in two ways: directly, by supporting nerve cell structure and function, and indirectly, by increasing the availability of nutrients to brain cells through improved circulation.

Studies investigating the evolution of human dietary patterns suggest that the human diet had a ratio of about one to one of omega-6 to omega-3 EFAs at least until the advent of agriculture. Unfortunately, our modern fast-food diet is extremely top-heavy in omega-6 vegetable oils, resulting in an unbalanced ten-to-one or higher ratio. Add to this the high amounts of saturated fats, trans fats, and nutrient-deficient foods present in the typical American diet, and it is clear why many people in the United States are overweight or obese and deficient in their levels of omega-3 fatty acids, which places them at high risk for chronic diseases during their later years. An unfavorable ratio—high omega-6 to low omega-3 EFA—can lead to increased inflammation throughout the body, which may be the leading culprit in the development of chronic diseases and, as you know, wrinkled, sagging skin.

Increasing the intake of omega-3 fatty acids and reducing omega-6 fatty acids may help prevent excessive inflammation by inhibiting the expression of a gene involved in the production of inflammatory-related proteins and help lessen the risk and/or progression of chronic diseases.

Unfortunately, it is often difficult for people to consume a diet that contains a favorable ratio of essential fatty acids, since much of our food supply is heavily skewed toward fast foods, dairy products, and meat, which are high in omega-6 fatty acids and low in omega-3 fatty acids. It's time for me to make a point about meat. We have been told that red meat has an unhealthy nutrient profile. This is true if we are talking about agribusiness and grain-fed cattle raised on feedlots. If you have access to 100 percent grass-fed, pasture-raised beef and lamb, the nutrient profile begins to resemble that of cold-water fish. Grass-fed beef and lamb contain high levels of omega-3 and conjugated linoleic acid, making this type of meat a healthy choice.

The good news is that people are becoming more aware of and receptive to the value of adding more plant-based foods including fruits, vegetables, seeds, nuts, and legumes to their diets. Not only will this help increase the intake of omega-3 fatty acids and shift the balance back to a favorable, noninflammatory ratio of omega-6 to omega-3 EFAs, but eating more plant-based foods will improve a person's antioxidant and overall nutritional status. Increasing the amount of omega-3 EFAs while decreasing omega-6 EFAs in the diet can help control inflammation, support cardiovascular and neurological function, promote tissue repair and rejuvenation, and may also help regulate cholesterol, sugar levels, and blood pressure, all of which lower the risk of chronic disease and enhance vitality.

Conversion of ALA into EPA and DHA

Two of the richest vegetarian sources of ALA are chia seeds and flaxseeds. The primary long-chain omega-3 fatty acid is DHA. The richest sources of DHA are marine algae, marine plankton, and the fish that consume them (salmon, sardines, and so on). The main sources of DHA in the diet are fish and fish oils, although recently, vegetarian supplements using DHA extracted from marine algae have been introduced to the marketplace.

ALA is directly involved in promoting health even though most of the benefits of omega-3 intake are attributed to the omega-3 long-chain fatty acids eicosapentaenoic acid (EPA) and docosahexaenoic acid (DHA), of which ALA is a precursor. Though the conversion of these two omega-3 fatty acids from ALA is generally considered relatively slow and inefficient, a plant-based diet with a higher level of ALA than LA may be sufficient to maintain adequate levels of both EPA and DHA.

Since EPA and DHA are present mainly in fish and absent in land-based food, it is generally assumed that sufficient levels of EPA and DHA in the body can be achieved only by consuming fish or fish oil supplements. Evidence actually suggests otherwise. Since a substantial percentage of people throughout human history have not been coastal dwellers and therefore have had to rely on land-based foods rather than on a diet including fish, it is reasonable to assume that their omega-3 intake has been almost exclusively in the form of ALA and not EPA or DHA. It follows that since EPA and DHA are both necessary for optimal health, adequate amounts of EPA and DHA must be produced from ALA, since it is the only source of omega-3 fatty acids in the diet for noncoastal-dwelling humans. If direct consumption of EPA and DHA were necessary for maintaining adequate levels of these two long-chain omega-3 fatty acids in the body, all humans would have had to eat fish in order just to survive, but this is obviously not the case. It seems reasonable that eating a diet rich in ALA should provide sufficient levels of EPA and DHA in our bodies for proper growth, development, and overall health. A diet that includes the right amount of ALA in a favorable ratio to omega-6 fatty acids should provide enough EPA and DHA to maintain health.

One study demonstrated that women are capable of converting substantial percentages of dietary ALA into the long-chain omega-3 fatty acids EPA (21%), DPA (6%), and DHA (9%), while a similar study of men found that ALA was converted into EPA (8%) and DPA (8%) but not into detectable levels of DHA. Since synthesized DHA can remain in the body for up to a week, it may not be necessary to produce high levels of it on a day-to-day basis.

A recent study indicates that recommendations for DHA supplementation of more than 1,000 milligrams may actually be excessive, since only about 200 milligrams of DHA consumed each day for two weeks were required to produce a beneficial antioxidant effect. The highest dose given, 1,600 milligrams per day, was associated with increased oxidative stress in the body. This oxidative stress may have resulted from having insufficient antioxidants in the body to protect the higher levels of circulating fatty acids from oxidation.

Though consuming fish or fish oil supplements has been considered the most reliable and convenient way to obtain EPA and DHA, it may not be the only solution, but it is still the best choice, because the body doesn't have to convert fish or fish oil to an active form. **As a vegetable source of omega-3 fatty acids, chia seeds are unsurpassed, even by flaxseeds.** Though supplementing the diet with modest amounts of high-quality, toxin-free fish oils is beneficial, increasing the intake of ALA from vegetable sources such as chia seeds while decreasing the consumption of fast foods containing high levels of omega-6 fatty acids will also help supply the body with the proper levels of health-promoting omega-3 fatty acids. Organic chia seeds can be valuable in helping to achieve a desirable fatty-acid balance for optimal health and longevity.

Leptin and Weight Loss

Health professionals, myself included, agree that reducing caloric intake in the form of high-glycemic carbohydrates and eating healthful fats and high-quality (high-protein-efficiency-ratio) protein, in conjunction with increasing daily exercise levels, are the keys to weight loss. However, there are other factors that may play critical roles in whether a weight loss program is successful as well as safe.

As any desperate dieter knows, the body is far more efficient at storing fat than burning it. Chronic dieters find that with each new diet, they gain back the lost weight faster, and losing weight becomes more difficult. One explanation of this metabolic phenomenon involves the action of a protein called leptin.

Leptin is produced in fat cells. It is released into the blood, in which it then travels to the brain and other peripheral tissues that are involved in regulating appetite and energy balance. As fat cells accumulate more fat, more leptin is produced and released into the blood, signaling the brain to curb appetite.

Obese people produce greater amounts of leptin per fat cell, which might sound like good news but is not. Rather than causing a decrease in appetite, chronic high levels of leptin may lead to the desensitization of the leptin receptors, making them resistant to its appetite-suppressing effects. There is a reason why obese people often feel hungry all the time.

The fact that fat cells accumulate more fat is worth exploring at this point.

Fat as an Endocrine Organ

Scientists have discovered an alarming characteristic of fat cells—one that was not known until quite recently. We now know that body fat, known scientifically as white adipose tissue, is not an inert deposit of fat cells, stored in the body as a result of overeating. Fat cells are anything *but* inert. They function as a highly active endocrine organ.

Body fat is an agglomeration of cells that communicate with other organ systems, including the brain, liver, bone marrow, adrenal cortex, skeletal muscle, sympathetic nervous system, and immune system. In addition, body fat produces hormones, as do the organs that make up the endocrine system: the pancreas, thyroid, parathyroid, adrenals, pineal, pituitary, and testes or ovaries.

This is extremely important because it means that the body fat itself controls how much body fat is stored. Our energy expenditure, appetite, and immune system are also affected because our body fat adipokines, hormones that the body secretes, are proteins that act as messengers in the body. A type of cytokine, cell-to-cell signaling protein, adipokines can be pro-inflammatory, contributing to chronic, systemic, subclinical inflammation.

This means that the greater the amount of body fat, the more inflammation is generated. The presence of a large amount of body fat causes the fat cells to secrete a nourishing cocktail of growth factors that promote new blood vessel growth to feed the accumulation of fat. However, the blood vessel growth cannot keep pace with the fast-growing mass of fat cells, so the fat cells become oxygen-starved. These oxygen-starved cells then start releasing inflammatory chemicals to further trigger blood vessel growth. As you can see, this mass of fat cells, which is now functioning as an active endocrine organ, is far more than just an aesthetic/cosmetic problem; fat sends destructive, pro-inflammatory signals to every organ system in the body. To sum up how fat makes us fatter, consider these points:

- People with excess weight have increased inflammation.
- This inflammation interferes with the ability to utilize insulin and blood sugar for energy (NF-κB blocks insulin).
- This leads to the storage of fat.
- Stored fat cells function as an endocrine organ, creating even more inflammatory chemicals.
- This leads to increased inflammation.
- The increased inflammation inhibits insulin and energy usage and causes the accumulation of additional excess fat.

When fat stores are diminished during reduced caloric intake, leptin levels fall and appetite increases. The problem for dieters is that increased leptin levels have much less of an effect on appetite than do decreased leptin levels. Dieting causes decreased leptin blood levels, which are accompanied not only by continual food cravings but also by reduced thermogenesis (fat metabolism) unless key metabolic nutrients, such as those in the Metabolic Miracle diet, are supplemented by the body. This is thought to be an adaptive response to conserve body fat to protect against famine. This situation makes losing weight more difficult as a diet progresses, leading to a "hitting the wall" phenomenon, or the inability to lose additional weight.

The Metabolic Miracle

One of the most pressing and important issues in aging is the progressive weight gain and muscle loss described in the discussion of sarcopenia.

After years of working with many patients who were struggling unsuccessfully to lose excess weight and keep it off, I concluded that the current weight loss regimens were ineffective at best and detrimental at worst. It was very disheartening to see, time and time again, a hard-won weight loss followed by the weight all being gained back—and then some!

The psychological aspects of this failure were profound and dispiriting. I needed to give these patients a completely new way of approaching weight loss, one that would keep them motivated, incentivized, and, most important, enthusiastically confident that they would achieve and maintain their goals safely.

I knew that the anti-inflammatory diet was both extremely effective and powerful, but I wanted more—I wanted a way to jump-start their weight loss while ensuring that their mental and physical well-being stayed intact. In addition, I wanted to maintain the incredible antiaging and beauty benefits that are associated with the anti-inflammatory diet. We have all observed friends, coworkers, and relatives who have lost a great deal of weight and are shocked to see their tired, haggard appearance, which makes them look years older, even as we try to compliment them on achieving their goal. As we learned earlier in this chapter, it is the bone and muscle loss caused by the vast majority of diets that is responsible for the aging effect. The Metabolic Miracle diet avoids this by ensuring that the body has more than adequate and highly bioavailable nutrients to protect muscle and bone while rapidly metabolizing body fat. The various nutrients in the anti-inflammatory Metabolic Miracle weight loss diet increase the sensitivity of all cell surface hormone receptors for insulin and leptin. The Metabolic Miracle diet resensitizes cells to hormones needed for appetite control and maintenance of muscle mass. Since the high-protein-efficiency-ratio meal replacement is rapidly absorbed, the appetite-suppressing nutrients reach the hypothalamus in a matter of minutes, suppressing appetite and relieving the sensation of hunger.

The concept of meal replacement drinks has long fascinated me. Many people have successfully lost weight using this method, although just as many have gained it all back. I knew that the concept was sound. The problem lay with the available options, all of which were grossly inadequate in terms of nutrition, satiety, and appetite control.

I was determined to help these individuals lose weight rapidly in a healthy manner yet not sacrifice the health benefits of my traditional anti-inflammatory diet. I was confident that by taking the anti-inflammatory approach, my patients could successfully preserve muscle tissue and bone while metabolizing body fat.

DEFINING OBESITY

Obesity has traditionally been defined as a weight at least 20 percent above the ideal weight corresponding to the lowest death rate for individuals of a specific height, gender, and age. A weight of 20 to 40 percent over ideal weight is considered mildly obese; 40 to 100 percent over ideal weight is considered moderately obese; and 100 percent over ideal weight is considered severely, or morbidly, obese.

The BMI (Body Mass Index)

Another way to determine healthy weight is via the body mass index (BMI). This number is calculated from a person's weight and height. BMI, as defined by the Centers for Disease Control and Prevention, is a fairly reliable indicator of body fat for most people. BMI does not measure body fat directly, but research has shown that it correlates well with direct measures of body fat, such as underwater weighing and dual-energy X-ray absorptiometry.

To calculate your BMI, see the directions at www.nhlbisupport .com/bmi.

Rising to the Challenge

The first challenge I faced in developing a metabolic meal replacement program was ensuring that high-quality protein, providing all of the essential amino acids, would be bioavailable. It must be able to be absorbed and utilized to enhance the immune system while nourishing and rebuilding the body on a cellular level. To meet these criteria, I needed a food that rated very high on a scale known as the protein efficiency ratio (PER). The PER is a measure of how much the amino acids will be absorbed after a particular food is eaten.

From 1919 until 1991, the PER was the gold standard of the U.S. government for evaluating the quality of protein in food. The PER is not commonly used today. Other methods (such as PDCAA, or Protein Digestibility Corrected Amino Acid Score, a biologic value that measures the protein retained after it has been absorbed) are sometimes used, but I don't believe they are as reliably accurate as the tried-and-true PER, which is extremely accurate and more precise than the newer method of rating proteins.

The PER became the cornerstone of the creation of a nourishing tool designed for rapid weight loss. When it was accompanied by a complete spectrum of metabolic enhancers, I was confident that I had the winning formula. I was particularly interested in trying this on several patients who were morbidly obese.

The next step was identifying the ideal source of protein. Albumin is the single most abundant protein found in the serum portion of our blood. When measured by laboratory tests, the presence of albumin is a strong indicator of the overall health of an individual. A wonderful and widely available food source of albumin is egg whites.

When we think of high-quality protein, we tend to think of a big steak or another animal source of protein such as chicken or turkey. But even these high-protein sources result in a PER that doesn't equal that of uncooked egg white albumin, whose PER or biologic value is close to 100 percent. If that same egg white is cooked, cross-linking of the proteins takes place and the PER drops considerably, by about 20 to 30 percent.

I was eager to explore the use of pure, organic, pasteurized egg white–sourced albumin with such an outstanding PER for a weight loss program. My notion was to create a Metabolic Miracle Meal Replacement that would satisfy hunger and accelerate weight loss.

Another supernutrient had to be part of the meal replacement. From my own experience with organic virgin coconut oil, I knew I had found my metabolic booster.

Organic Virgin Coconut Oil: The Saturated Fat You Should Eat Every Day

Coconut oil is a superfood I have incorporated into my own diet. I am certain you have heard the dire warnings about saturated fats, but they are not to be confused with the trans fats in processed foods. Saturated fats constitute 50 percent of our cells' membranes, the phospholipid component of every cell. They strengthen the cell walls, protecting the inside of the cell. They play a vital role in the health of our bones, protect the liver from alcohol and other toxins, and ensure the proper use of the omega-3 fatty acids.

Virgin coconut oil is a medium-chain saturated fat (MCFA) that speeds weight loss, lowers cholesterol, reduces the risk of heart attacks, and improves diabetic conditions. MCFAs do not need the liver and gallbladder to digest them, which means instant energy and increased metabolic rate through thermogenesis. Coconut oil is beneficial to the immune system, because it has antimicrobial and antifungal properties. Coconut oil targets the thyroid and beefs up the metabolism, melting abdominal fat quickly. I knew I had to include this powerful nutrient in my weight loss program.

The Metabolic Miracle Meal Replacement

I wanted to use these ingredients—egg white–sourced albumin and virgin coconut oil—as a Metabolic Miracle Meal Replacement, which I carefully balanced with nutritional supplements that act as mitochondrial metabolic enhancers, cell membrane stabilizers, insulin sensitizers, and blood sugar stabilizers.

To ensure that your Metabolic Miracle Meal Replacement drink is rich in nutrients and flavor, I recommend these recipes:

- Puree ⅓ cup of blueberries, raspberries, or mixed berries of your choice in a blender.

  or

- Mix 1 teaspoon of non-Dutch-processed cocoa with stevia and a little hot water. Blend until thoroughly smooth.
- Add 1 teaspoon of organic virgin coconut oil to either the berries or the cocoa and blend until smooth.
- Add the protein and stir. Do not blend, as this will make the drink too foamy. For women approximately five feet, four inches tall with moderate activity, I suggest 6 ounces of the protein source in liquid form or as labeled if it is in powdered form.
- Take one packet of the Metabolic Formula Supplement, available on my Web site in convenient packets of capsules, or create your own by referring to the list opposite.

The Metabolic Formula Supplement

My selections for the nutrients in the Metabolic Formula Supplement packets were based on years of published research on their efficacy in regulating metabolism and body weight. As always, taking a high-quality multivitamin is important. I have discussed the other nutrients at length in the previous chapters, but list them and their functions here as a quick reference as well:

- Co Q10 and carnitine—work in the mitochondria to enhance energy production and efficiently convert food into energy so that it is not stored as body fat
- Omega-3 essential fatty acids—assist in converting food into energy rather than storing it, while keeping cell membranes flexible and supple so that insulin receptors are sensitive
- Glutamine—an amino acid that helps control carbohydrate cravings among other benefits
- Niacin-bound chromium (NBC)—stabilizes blood sugar and aids in cell membrane function
- Conjugated linoleic acid (CLA)—stabilizes blood sugar and aids in cell membrane function
- Curcumin gel capsule—provides all the many benefits of turmeric

Before undertaking any new dietary or supplemental program, you need to consult with your health care provider.

The Metabolic Miracle Diet

I started a number of my patients with the Metabolic Miracle Meal Replacement and the Metabolic Formula Supplement as their first meal of the day. The results were more positive than I could possibly have anticipated. Each patient's protein needs were carefully calculated based on his or her muscle mass, activity levels, and gender. Within four to five minutes of taking the meal replacement drink all individuals reported a feeling of satiety. This high level of appetite satisfaction lasted for several hours. They also reported a lift in their energy levels. Note that this appetite control fails without the presence of the metabolic nutrients.

I then repeated the same formula (meal replacement drink along with the metabolic supplement formula) for their second meal of the day. In the evening, each patient enjoyed a meal of the standard Perricone anti-inflammatory diet. This consisted of the following:

- Six ounces of grilled salmon on a bed of 2 ounces of cooked lentils
- A watercress salad dressed with olive oil and lemon juice or vinegar
- One cup of steamed broccoli

In addition, the metabolic supplement formula was administered at this regular meal. I also encouraged my patients to drink eight 8-ounce glasses of fresh spring water per day and to switch from coffee to green tea. I also instructed the patients to have a 3- to 4-ounce serving of the meal replacement drink as a snack if they became hungry or felt their energy levels ebbing.

The clinical results I observed with patients using the two high-PER meal replacements and the one regular meal in conjunction with the Metabolic Formula were dramatic. In two weeks, the average weight loss was 12 pounds in individuals who were carrying an extra 25 pounds of body fat. After one month on the meal replacement program, the average weight loss was 18 to 22 pounds. Most dramatic was the weight loss in those who were morbidly obese, with several patients losing close to 150 pounds during a four- to six-month period.

Most important, the individuals participating in the program lost body fat and maintained their lean muscle mass. All appeared vibrant, radiant, energetic, and remarkably younger-looking upon completion of the program.

The majority of individuals continued taking the Metabolic Supplement Formula with regular meals, even after reaching their goal, to maintain their weight loss and new level of vibrant energy. The majority also continued with one meal replacement per day as a lifestyle change, because it made it that much easier to maintain their goal weight.

The Metabolic Miracle Meal Replacement formula is also a great safety net against the overeating we tend to indulge in during holidays, celebrations, and vacations. By replacing two meals per day after such indulgence, we can be sure to keep unwanted body fat at bay and maintain our new healthy weight.

Two aspects of the Metabolic Miracle diet are important secrets of its success; one is psychological and the other is physiological.

The psychological advantage is knowing that at two of three meals a day, optimum nutrients are delivered quickly and efficiently, with complete regulation of the appetite mechanism. We are not tempted to fall off the wagon and binge on junk foods, because our appetite and mood are stabilized.

The physiological advantage of the high PER rating results from the rapid changes in the gut affecting the hypothalamic appetite mechanism within minutes of ingestion. The appetite is satisfied, yet the blood sugar and insulin remain low, releasing the lock on body fat.

Kelly's Story

I first met Kelly in the greenroom of a popular network morning show. I was appearing to promote my new book, and she was going on to discuss her new sitcom. The greenroom atmosphere is always pleasant and upbeat. Guests are both nervous and excited, producers and junior producers are constantly running in and out, and long tables are filled with delicious foods such as fresh fruit, raw vegetables, cheeses, and yogurt, as well as a mind-boggling variety of pastries and muffins. As I was helping myself to a bowl of berries, Kelly, whose plate held a large cheese Danish, turned and said, "Dr. Perricone, I am so excited to meet you." As we headed to a private seating area with a stupendous view of one of Manhattan's most iconic sights, Kelly confided her frustration with her weight. "I know, I know, I shouldn't be eating this stuff. Usually I am pretty good, but when I'm nervous I tend to self-medicate with sugary, starchy foods." A beautiful and hugely successful actress on both the big and small screens, Kelly was well known for her ongoing battles with the bulge—which unfortunately she appeared to be losing.

Losing weight is perhaps the greatest physical challenge healthy people face, and one of the hardest to overcome. "Kelly," I said, "believe it or not, successful weight loss is not rocket science. Losing weight is also not simply about cutting calories and exercising more."

"Amen to that!" Kelly exclaimed. "If I could just stop eating . . ."

"It's not even about that, Kelly," I explained. "What would you say if I could promise that you would lose body fat and inches rapidly, without feeling tired, hungry, or depressed? I can put you on a simple-to-follow program that turns on the genes that code for fat burning, and turns off the genes that store fat while preserving precious muscle mass and bone." This was particularly important for Kelly, as she was in her late forties and experiencing the loss of the bone-protective hormone estrogen.

Kelly and the Metabolic Miracle

The various nutrients in the anti-inflammatory Metabolic Miracle diet increase the sensitivity of all cell surface hormone receptors, including insulin and leptin. Making sure that the cells develop sensitivity to the hormones necessary to keep the appetite at bay and utilize body fat for energy, rather than storing it, while protecting muscle mass is the most important first step. I explained to Kelly that certain foods trigger an out-of-control appetite, especially as we get older. Years of eating the wrong foods result in a loss of sensitivity to insulin, which ends up causing swings in blood sugar, increased appetite, and weight gain.

To be successful, Kelly needed to stop eating the foods that would trigger this insulin response. I assured her that if her appetite was sated, her cravings would drop along with her weight.

Kelly was not particularly athletic, and she was showing signs of the sarcopenia described at the start of this chapter. I made a note to refer Kelly to Wini Linguvic, the esteemed celebrity trainer and yoga expert who contributed the yoga chapter for this book. I knew that nothing would get Kelly into great physical condition as quickly as the Metabolic Miracle diet combined with yoga—and without placing strain on her joints.

Getting Started

Since Kelly had a significant amount of weight to lose—60-plus pounds—I recommended that she replace two meals per day with the Metabolic Miracle Meal Replacement and supplements. This meal replacement drink would rapidly satisfy her hunger while suppressing her appetite for hours—all within a few minutes of ingestion. I also started Kelly on daily servings of chia seeds, which promote healthy weight loss, have an outstanding omega-3 profile, and have unique abilities to increase endurance and stamina.

Kelly needed a boost to her spirits and her energy levels—and chia seeds fit the bill. The omega-3s found in fish oil, chia seeds, and cold-water fish such as salmon and sardines can also uncouple oxidative phosphorylation, turning on fat burning and partitioning energy so that it is not stored as fat. Thus, essential fatty acids can affect gene expression by activating PPARs that turn on the fat-burning genes.

Perhaps the most important cease-and-desist order for Kelly to follow, if she wanted this plan to succeed, involved totally eliminating any food or beverage that contained high-fructose corn syrup (HFCS). I have talked and written about the obesity link and rapid weight gain associated with HFCS ingestion for years. I have also been confronted on numerous occasions by other health experts and scientists, who vehemently claim that there is no difference between sucrose, derived from sugarcane or beets, and high-fructose corn syrup.

An outstanding study recently released from Princeton put the nail in the coffin of that fallacy. Researchers there found that *not* all sweeteners are equal when it comes to weight gain. In this study, published in the journal *Pharmacology Biochemistry & Behavior*, researchers from the Department of Psychology and the Princeton Neuroscience Institute discovered that rats with access to high-fructose corn syrup piled on significantly more pounds than rats with access to table sugar, although their basic caloric intake was the same. The really bad news is that, in addition to their considerable weight gain, the rats eating the HFCS developed abnormal amounts of body fat, especially in the abdominal area. This abdominal body fat, also known as visceral or toxic fat, is the hardest to lose. These fat cells, which act as an endocrine organ in their own right, pour out a constant stream of toxic, pro-inflammatory messenger chemicals (cytokines) that threaten overall health and greatly lessen the prospects of successful weight control. Central obesity sets the stage for a host of health concerns such as heart disease, strokes, and diabetes. HFCS also significantly raises triglycerides.

To clarify, there are two types of fat: subcutaneous, found under the skin, and visceral, located in the abdomen and surrounding our vital organs. Visceral fat is extremely dangerous, as it is metabolized by the liver, which turns it into cholesterol that circulates in the blood. This is the so-called bad cholesterol, low-density lipoproteins, or LDLs, which collects in the arteries, forming plaque (deposits of fats, inflammatory cells, proteins, and calcium along the lining of arteries). The plaque builds up and narrows the artery, resulting in atherosclerosis.

"Some people have claimed that high-fructose corn syrup is no different than other sweeteners when it comes to weight gain and obesity, but our results make it clear that this just isn't true, at least under the conditions of our tests," said Princeton researcher and psychology professor Bart Hoebel, who specializes in the neuroscience of appetite, weight, and sugar addiction. "When rats are drinking high-fructose corn syrup at levels well below those in soda pop, they're becoming obese—every single one, across the board. Even when rats are fed a high-fat diet, you don't see this; they don't all gain extra weight."

The rats drinking HFCS in the Princeton study became obese and those drinking sugar water did not. In a classic example of gene expression, it appears that the fructose activated the genes that store fat, while the sucrose activated the genes that either process the glucose for energy or store it as a carbohydrate known as glycogen in the liver and muscles.

Tricking the Brain into Overeating

When we consume such simple sugars as HFCS, we cause an immediate pro-inflammatory spike in our blood sugar. Unlike glucose, however, fructose *does not* stimulate the secretion of insulin or enhance the production of leptin—key hormones that regulate the appetite. Since insulin and leptin act as signals to the brain for the regulation of food intake and body weight, the ability of fructose to circumvent these mechanisms may contribute to overeating. This completely upsets the body's natural balance. Fructose bypasses the natural mechanisms that prevent overeating and tricks the body into thinking it is still hungry—even after consuming a large meal—making it a fast-food marketer's dream! No wonder they supersize the sodas! (And those who drink them.)

The reason for this is the difference between the digestive and absorptive processes for glucose and fructose. When we consume large amounts of fructose, which is basically an unregulated source of fuel for the liver, it is converted to both fat and cholesterol. As my readers know, I am no advocate of sugar—in fact, *sugar is toxic*—but the effects of fructose, particularly in the form of high-fructose corn syrup, are an even more significant cause for alarm. I am not talking about the naturally occurring fructose found in fresh fruit. Eating fresh fruit provides us with many nutrients, minerals, enzymes, and phytochemicals, and is highly recommended.

The Metabolic Miracle Meal Replacement

Kelly, whose high-profile lifestyle and livelihood underscored the importance of looking good, was a perfect candidate for the Metabolic Miracle diet. For breakfast and lunch, she had the Metabolic Miracle Meal Replacement Drink and the recommended supplements. For dinner she had a piece of fresh fish—salmon as often as possible—or a boneless, skinless chicken breast sautéed lightly in olive oil and served on a bed of cooked lentils, together with a salad made of watercress and dressed with extra-virgin olive oil and fresh lemon juice and a cup of steamed veggies, such as broccoli or cauliflower. I also recommended that she drink a lot of green tea, which contains a very special catechin, EGCG, that accelerates weight loss and helps block fat absorption.

We must eat fat to burn fat, which means that cold-water fish, chia seeds, extra-virgin coconut oil, and olive oil all help us burn fat. The pro-inflammatory sugary, starchy foods are just the opposite. Because they raise insulin and blood sugar levels, they put an actual "lock" on fat burning. The Metabolic Miracle Meal Replacement, the supplements, and the recommended dinner menu consist of foods with potent anti-inflammatory properties as well as highly bioavailable nutrients that protected Kelly's muscle and bone while she rapidly metabolized body fat, ensuring that her weight loss would be rapid.

Within weeks, Kelly had lost 25 pounds and 5 inches from her waistline. "Dr. Perricone, I am going to stay on this forever!" she vowed enthusiastically at a follow-up meeting six weeks later. Eventually she would introduce more foods into her diet, but she planned to maintain the Metabolic Miracle Meal Replacement drink for breakfast, as it kept her energized and filled with a sense of well-being for hours. Kelly also intended to take the supplements on a regular basis, because they improved both her physical and mental well-being.

The high-quality protein in the Metabolic Miracle Meal Replacement drink is vital to cellular repair, and the metabolic supplements are critical to the suppression of appetite. This protein, as well as the omega-3 essential fats, will ensure that your skin will be radiant and glowing as the unwanted body fat melts away. For Kelly, whose face is her fortune, the results were superb—she looked years younger, with a luminous complexion to match her new lithe, slim, and toned figure.

Wini told me that Kelly was a wonderful yoga student, eager to learn and making rapid progress. Like nutrigenomics and the metabolic miracle, yoga is all about self-empowerment. As with nutrigenomics and the metabolic miracle, visible results are seen in a very short time, which helps to keep Kelly's enthusiasm and motivation at optimal levels.

I know the Metabolic Miracle diet plan will help you to take control of your weight and consequently your health. Being chronically overweight stresses our bodies and will age us prematurely. Following my program will help you to maintain a lean body at a healthy weight, increase your energy, and conquer your food cravings. You will lose weight without that haggard, dried-out, pale, and exhausted look. Instead, you will be radiant, fresh, and youthful in body and spirit.

Chapter Four

NOVEL TOPICAL AND NUTRITIONAL

STRATEGIES TO RENEW, REPAIR,

AND REJUVENATE

You cannot stop the clock; it ticks incessantly. But you can slow down the aging process that goes along with that ticking clock—an important goal for Forever Young. The key to aging, in its simplest terms, is cell damage and the reduced ability of our bodies to repair or replace damaged cells. The logical first step, then, is to protect the cell before damage occurs, including the cell membrane, mitochondria, and DNA, as well as the downregulation of inflammatory genes. A strategy of the first defense is usually the best defense. There may be no turning back the clock, but aging can occur gracefully, extending the years of vitality, health, and beauty.

As you will learn in this chapter, there is a very special and unique group of foods that can provide us with the perfect tools. Most important, you will learn that true beauty is radiant health, and this chapter will give you the tools to achieve this goal.

However, I want to start this chapter with one of my most exciting discoveries in topical skin treatments. As so often happens, the inspiration came about as far from my office as one can get.

As a scientist and inventor, many of my happiest hours are spent in the lab, researching strategies for healthy aging and youthful skin. Other fields draw my attention, particularly the aerospace industry. I have always loved flying my own plane. This passion has led to my research in developing various technologies for increasing safety and energy efficiency in aircraft. As I pursued this interest in jet propulsion systems and fuel economy, I became fascinated with the concept of space.

I have had the good fortune to work with scientists at Los Alamos National Laboratories. Under a special arrangement with the National Laboratories known as a cooperative research and development agreement (CRADA), my company began working with the top plasma physicists in the world. At Los Alamos, we worked with devices that could separate electrons from nuclei, creating plasma gas at room temperatures, instead of the several-thousand-degree centigrade temperatures normally seen in a plasma cloud. The key was to create a powerful electric field that would separate the electrons from the nucleus without creating heat, a process known as cold-plasma technology. This process inspired me to create a revolutionary new concept for delivering nutrients to the skin.

Cold-Plasma Technology

Picture space, an empty universe, as a carrier. This space is made up of approximately 99 percent plasma, charged particles floating through space.

Plasma Facts

- Plasma makes up 99 percent of the universe.
- Plasma is not a gas, a liquid, or a solid; it is a different form of matter. Plasma is an electrically charged cloud.

- This cloud arises when the positively charged nuclei of the atom separate from the electrons.
- This normally occurs at very high temperatures of thousands of degrees because high temperatures are required to separate the electrons from the nucleus of the atom (protons and neutrons).
- Physicists have learned how to create plasma at low temperatures (cold plasma), and this has opened the door to thousands of applications.

The recognition that plasma exists in a carrier, such as space, in this instance as an *ionic suspension*, gave me the idea of creating an ionic suspension as a special carrier system for topical application. Just as the plasma in space provides all the building materials necessary to create the planets and the stars, I planned to create what I would later name Cold Plasma, an ionic suspension system in a jar: a carrier full of charged particles.

Ionic Suspension

If you are wondering why I would create a carrier system capable of delivering charged particles to the skin, consider this fact: many of the highly important nutrients that are needed by the cell either carry an electric charge and/or are very large molecules, making it difficult or impossible for them to benefit the skin. A common problem in delivering highly active particles with electrical charges to the cells is that charged particles clump or aggregate together, falling out of the solution.

Another problem is that charged particles do not readily penetrate skin or cells because the charge itself prevents movement of the ion, whether into the layers of the skin or through the cell plasma membrane. In this special patented proprietary carrier system, these ions are insulated, allowing them to rapidly move through barriers that can normally not be traversed. There are certain nutrients that are needed by the skin to produce the matrix of collagen and elastin that is absolutely necessary to youthful skin. Of particular importance are the *glycosaminoglycans,* which are the precursors of collagen. Higher levels of glycosaminoglycans are evidence of new collagen production in the skin.

It has long been a goal of scientists working in dermatology to find methods of increasing levels of the glycosaminoglycans in the skin, to create a more youthful appearance by building up the underlying matrix. The impairment of glycosaminoglycan synthesis is what results in much of the damage to and destruction of aged skin.

Scientists were delighted to discover that long-term use of alpha-hydroxy acids with concentrations between 10 and 20 percent showed a marked increase in glycosaminoglycan levels in the skin. Even better, powerful pharmaceuticals such as growth hormones (epidermal growth factor) have resulted in an 80 percent increase in the production of glycosaminoglycans. My research has progressed significantly further and allowed me to develop a system in which I can deliver vital nutrients in an ionic form (charged particles) that increase glycosaminoglycan production by *more than 150 percent* in a completely safe and physiological manner—without having to use powerful hormones like epidermal growth factor. This ionic suspension can be the catalyst that will renew the vital matrix and keep our skin youthful into advanced years.

The use of this new, patented proprietary delivery system acts as both an incredible insulator and a carrier, allowing it to carry charged particles by preventing them from aggregating or precipitating together and falling out of the solution. They stay in the solution, where they belong, and do not end up just sitting at the bottom of the jar.

The same ionic suspension proprietary carrier system that insulates and carries these molecules in the suspension also ensures that they can be of the greatest benefit to the skin, resulting in a significantly firmer and smoother appearance.

Vitamin B3 for Superior Cell Protection

Vitamin B3 is one of eight B vitamins. It is also known as niacin (nicotinic acid) and has two other forms, niacinamide (nicotinamide) and inositol hexanicotinate.

The nicotinamide form of vitamin B3 is an extremely powerful cell protectant and can prevent damage to DNA. It is protective of all organ systems and can prevent the cognitive decline resulting from aging and Alzheimer's disease. Nicotinamide is also protective of blood vessels, preventing inflammation and subsequent atherosclerosis. It also delays the onset and progress of diabetes.

This cell-protective agent functions on a mitochondrial level to prevent apoptosis (programmed cell death), thus saving brain cells, pancreatic cells, blood vessels, and other vital organ systems. Nicotinamide's powerful anti-inflammatory effects block pro-inflammatory cytokines that, in turn, block the progression of multiple disease processes, including multiple sclerosis, arthritis, and autoimmune diseases.

Nicotinamide also stabilizes blood sugar and prevents insulin resistance. This B vitamin also participates in energy production in the mitochondria. It maintains the integrity of the mitochondrial membrane, preventing the changes seen with aging. The most dramatic positive effects are seen in its ability to protect the genomic DNA from the degradation that is seen with aging and disease.

Through multiple mechanisms, such as the anti-inflammatory capability as well as protection of the mitochondria and DNA, niacinamide significantly increases cell longevity. The powerful cell-protective action of this single agent holds tremendous potential for both life extension and the prevention of *all* age-related diseases.

The Magic of Microcurrent

I am a huge fan of microcurrent treatments, which should be used regularly as a component of a healthful beauty regimen. Microcurrent is widely available in spas as well as in a new handheld machine that delivers wonderful benefits to the skin (see Resources section). As it is as easy to perform as applying your daily makeup, microcurrent is the perfect home treatment that can be done in a few minutes each day. The results are cumulative—in other words, they get better and better, just as going to the gym on a regular basis improves your body's muscle tone. A simple ten-minute daily regimen that alternates among the chin, cheeks, eyes, and forehead provides each area with optimal benefits.

Unlike exfoliating machines and other products, which can damage the skin over time, there are no long-term adverse effects associated with microcurrent. In fact, microcurrent is extremely therapeutic.

Once available only in spas, this treatment can be done at home. There is no difference between the power used in a home care system and that used in a professional machine. Microcurrent utilizes a subsensory electric current to reeducate the facial muscles while improving both the tone and the texture of the skin. The process diminishes the appearance of lines and wrinkles and produces a *natural lift* without the use of surgery or other invasive methods. When combined with powerful anti-inflammatory topicals and substances that help reverse the damage caused by aging, poor diet, stress, and the environment, it is a very holistic and natural approach to eliminating many of the unwelcome signs of aging.

Microcurrent facial treatments have been available in spas since the 1980s. They have been extremely popular in Europe and are now gaining ground in the United States as spas seek to attract the Botox consumer. The current catchphrase in the spa world is "results-oriented treatments." This represents a shift away from facials that pamper but do little to create meaningful improvement in a client's appearance, and it is an alternative to the minimally invasive medical treatments that have come to dominate the market in the last few years.

Minimally invasive medical treatments have grown dramatically in popularity since 2000 and have become a socially acceptable method of addressing the signs of aging. The attractions of these types of treatments are:

- The immediate and natural results they produce
- Their relative safety
- The fact that they can be done quickly via injection and without surgery
- Their affordability as compared with surgical procedures

The most popular among these minimally invasive procedures are Botox and hyaluronic acid fillers. Botox is botulinum toxin, a neurotoxic protein that works to relax the contraction of muscles by blocking nerve impulses. The result is muscles that can no longer contract, so the wrinkles they produce relax and soften. Hyaluronic acid treatments (marketed under trade names such as Restylane and Juvéderm) consist of injections of a hyaluronic acid gel into the dermis. Once administered, the gel joins to the dermal tissue and begins to bind the water molecules, which softens lines and smoothes out wrinkles. According to the American Society of Plastic Surgeons, its members performed more than five million Botox treatments in 2008 at an average price of $391 and more than one million hyaluronic acid filler injections at an average price of $578. Botox treatments have increased by 537 percent since 2000, and minimally invasive procedures have increased by 5 percent as a category over the last year despite some of the worst economic conditions in recent memory.

A somewhat alarming trend is that both women and men feel driven to start serious (and often very costly) surgical procedures at a younger and younger age. New fillers designed to plump up facial lines are being rushed to market and intensively advertised. The use of neurotoxins (neuro for "nerve," toxin for "poison") that paralyze muscles to smooth out wrinkles and expression lines is counterintuitive. When we lose muscle mass and tone, we lose the youthful contours of our face and body. The ultimate weak muscle is one that is paralyzed. That fact should lead one to conclude that paralyzing the muscles in the face may not be the best strategy for achieving a youthful look over the years that follow. Though these products offer a quick fix, what will be the long-term result?

I believe that there will always be a place for a wide variety of procedures, both surgical and nonsurgical, but I do not believe that the future of youthful-looking skin lies in an acceleration of invasive treatments, injectible fillers, neurotoxins, or radical surgery. **Great breakthroughs are being made in which safe yet genuinely transformative methodologies not only help restore damaged, aging skin to youthful suppleness but reinvigorate the entire body as well. Microcurrent is a key player in this movement.**

The new "Botox standard" of immediate results has challenged traditional spas as they look to fill the demand for these types of services while staying nonmedical. The result has been a movement on the part of spas to a combination of more cosmeceutical skin care products and the use of more advanced aesthetic equipment in their treatments. Microcurrent treatments are uniquely suitable because they are nonmedical and create improvements in the client's appearance that cannot be achieved by any of the medical procedures currently being offered.

There are great medical procedures for removing pigmented spots by means of laser, addressing wrinkles by filling them in or freezing the underlying muscle, and taking care of sagging skin by pulling it tighter through surgery. None of these procedures improves the underlying facial muscles. These muscles are unique in that they are attached to the skin, whereas other muscles are attached to the bones by tendons, so they have a profound impact on our appearance. As we age, the muscles in our face give in to the effects of gravity and underuse by drooping and causing a saggy appearance. Other muscles of the face—those on the forehead and around the eyes, for example—become contracted due to overuse and cause lines and wrinkles. Improving the underlying facial musculature has a direct impact on youthful appearance.

Microcurrent is unique in its ability to improve the muscles of the face to create a more youthful and toned appearance through a process that has come to be known as a nonsurgical face-lift. The treatments work on the muscles of the face through a combination of manual manipulation and biostimulation. Manual manipulation of the muscle is achieved through the use of two probes that gently massage the muscle along its origin and insertion points. The origin point of the muscle is the bone and the insertion point is where the muscle connects to the skin. Stimulating the muscle fibers at the origin and insertion points of the muscles involved gently coaxes them to stretch or shorten with no pain to the client. An atrophied muscle can be shortened and toned. A muscle in contraction can be stretched. This process, known as muscle reeducation, is the cornerstone of microcurrent facial treatments. The two-hand design allows the user to manipulate the muscle along these points while stimulating the entire length with microcurrent. Simply applying microcurrent to the face in a static manner will have the same biostimulation effects on the tissue but will lack the muscle reeducation benefits found in the proper treatments. This is an easy, pain-free treatment with long-lasting visible results—unlike the so-called quick fixes.

While mechanical stimulation of the muscle can be achieved through massage, microcurrent generates profound results through the simultaneous biostimulation of the muscle and surrounding tissue. One of the most notable benefits of microcurrent is its ability to improve the production of ATP, the chemical fuel in muscles that provides the energy they require to hold their position after being manipulated. As we learned in chapter 3, ATP is the primary energy currency in the body and powers virtually every activity of the cell and organism. Studies have shown that the application of microcurrent can increase the production of ATP by an astounding 500 percent. Microcurrent also helps correct the alignment of the muscle by communicating with the Golgi tendon organ (GTO). The GTO is a type of proprioceptor, a special nerve ending in the muscles and tendons and other organs that respond to stimuli regarding the position and movement of the body, that provides information about changes in muscle tension. At the same time that microcurrent works on the muscles, it also stimulates the underlying processes involved in promoting healthy skin. Specifically, its low levels of electricity have been shown to increase:

- Membrane active transport, critical to delivering nutrients intracellularly and exporting metabolic wastes extracellularly
- Protein synthesis, vital for tissue repair and regeneration
- Collagen production and thickness
- Elastin production
- Circulation

Microcurrent treatments are uniquely suited to a home care regimen because they produce immediate results that continue to improve with subsequent treatments. The ongoing improvement experienced with the application of these treatments has to do with the continued improvements in the underlying processes that keep the skin healthy, such as circulation and the production of collagen and elastin, as well as the continued improvements in ATP production.

It helps to view microcurrent treatments in the same way we view exercising the body. People who go to the gym and exercise once may see an improvement in the appearance of their muscles, but in a short period of time the results will go away if the muscles are not exercised again. On the other hand, someone who exercises consistently for a year can take a month off without losing the benefits achieved. Consistency is key.

This same principle applies to microcurrent treatments. Initially treatments should be performed in a series, followed by regular maintenance treatments. The first time a microcurrent treatment is done, the ATP in the muscles will be increased and then return to baseline levels shortly afterward. If ATP production is stimulated by another treatment shortly after the first, the levels remain high. The more treatments that are performed, the longer the ATP will remain stored in the muscle. Since ATP can be stockpiled and stored, treatment results are cumulative and become more effective as the series progresses. As the baseline ATP levels increase, the muscles will hold their tone longer.

Microcurrent is an extremely low level of electricity that mimics the electricity that naturally flows through our body. The primary function of microcurrent treatments is to stimulate the body's own healing processes to improve the skin and muscles of the face. The results are both natural and predictable, because the treatments work to restore the natural contours of our face and work within our own facial structure. The benefit of this is that the treatments will never produce a "bad face-lift" result. The effects will mimic your younger facial contours naturally, while increasing skin radiance thanks to increased blood circulation. Microcurrent, by definition, is one millionth of an amp of electricity. This extremely low level of electricity generally causes little to no sensation when applied to the face. Typical sensations may include a metallic taste in the mouth, lights flashing in the eyes, small muscle twitches when working around the eyes, and a tapping sensation felt on the back of the head when working on the forehead. One benefit of microcurrent treatments is an increase in blood flow to the area, which can appear as a slight reddening of the treated areas that typically goes away within a few minutes.

Most people experience results after a single microcurrent session, whether it is a softening of fine lines, a raising of the eyebrows, or even a profound lift to the cheeks. The treatment is great for any skin type, and recent research has shown that 100 percent of the people who tried a series of treatments reported seeing an improvement in their appearance. **The best results are seen after a series of microcurrent treatments is performed, with treatment frequency averaging four times per week for a month.**

For some people the term "microcurrent muscle stimulation" conjures up an image of electrodes attached to the face with the muscles contorting under the stimulation of a strong electrical current. Microcurrent is actually a very small amount of electricity applied to the facial muscles through probes that massage the muscles into a more natural position. The process is extremely comfortable, and there is no visible muscle contraction. In fact, the currents generally create little to no sensation at all.

Microcurrent treatments are ideal for home use because:

- Microcurrent is pain-free and very relaxing.
- The best results are achieved over time with regular treatments.
- The technique is simple and easy to perform while looking in the mirror.
- Quick ten-minute treatments may be performed to spot-treat problem areas.
- The treatment presents very few risks, even when compared with other home care products.
- Immediate results mean you can perform a treatment prior to a special occasion for a quick lift.
- Treatments can be performed daily.
- The results are natural and predictable.
- Spa treatments can be expensive.

Microcurrent benefits include:

- Production of ATP
- Production of elastin
- Production of collagen
- Tissue oxygenation
- Increased blood circulation
- Ion exchange
- Absorption of nutrients
- Elimination of waste products

Types of Microcurrent Treatments

EYES   The eyes are surrounded by a network of fine, narrow muscles that can become contracted and cause wrinkles from overuse. Microcurrent treatments stretch the lines at the corners of the eyes to reduce their appearance while lifting the eyebrow area. The muscles that cause the lines between the eyes are also treated in a stretching motion to help them release, while the muscles directly under the eyes are contracted to reduce sagging while firming the skin.

FOREHEAD   The vertical muscles that support the skin of the forehead have the primary function of lifting the eyebrows and are also used when a view is distant or dim. When these muscles are overused, they become shorter and create deep wrinkles. Microcurrent treatment of this area is used to stimulate the blood vessels for proper irrigation of the epidermis and to release the fontalis muscles from spasm to soften horizontal lines across the forehead.

CREASES AROUND THE MOUTH   The muscles that form the area around the mouth generally work in a downward fashion that can form vertical creases around the mouth. With microcurrent the muscles can be worked in an upward direction that lifts the area and progressively reduces wrinkles.

SAGGING CHIN   Chewing works the muscles in the jaw but does not stimulate the ones that correct sagging in the chin. The muscles tend to become elongated from underuse, causing the area to droop or sag. Microcurrent treatments cause these muscles to contract and tighten up any slackness under the chin. The effects are even more dramatic when combined with a new treatment called topical "Sub-D," which helps to rapidly firm the chin and jawline.

COMPLEXION   Regular use of microcurrent improves the underlying processes that support healthy skin, including collagen and elastin production, circulation of oxygenated blood, and the exchange of nutrients and waste products within the cells.

We have discussed rejuvenation from the outside by the use of Cold Plasma and microcurrent. We will now turn our attention to special foods and nutrients that are known to heal and restore, helping you to stay Forever Young.

Keep on the Grass

I am a huge fan of the "green foods," the young grasses of barley, wheat, rye, and oats before the grass is converted into grain. I recently had the opportunity to spend time with Bob Terry, Ph.D., a technical service adviser at Green Foods Corporation, to get the latest updates on the superb nutritional properties of green foods. A tremendous resource, Bob has generously shared important scientific data on how these nutrients both protect and rejuvenate our bodies at a cellular level—and, in the case of chia seeds (discussed in chapter 3), significantly increase our vitality, endurance, and energy. **A young cell is characterized by its energy, and with the cellular reenergizing that occurs with both the green foods and chia seeds, we may have a genuine Forever Young strategy that will work for all.**

For centuries these cereal grasses have been grown for their grains, which when ground are the main types of flour used in breads and other baked products. However, the gluten present in most grains, especially wheat, can be problematic. In fact, about 1 person in 133 has an allergy to gluten. After decades in practice, I observed that many of my patients had very low-grade or subclinical chronic inflammation and fatigue that were attributable to eating foods that are pro-inflammatory, for example, gluten-rich grains, especially wheat. In addition, many of them had a wheat or gluten allergy without knowing it. This does not mean that cereal grasses need to be avoided. The secret lies in harvesting and processing them before they begin to turn to grain. Once they convert to grain there is a sharp decline in the chlorophyll, protein, and vitamin content in conjunction with an increase in the level of cellulose (indigestible fiber).

I was giving a lecture at the American College of Nutrition Annual Symposium and invited Dr. Mark Hyman to participate in my seminar. In his lecture, he discussed the dangers of gluten for the general population—even those who don't have a gluten allergy or intolerance—because of its pro-inflammatory properties. Dr. Hyman explained that a protein in gluten is nearly identical to a substance that is part of the membrane structure of neurons in the brain. He stated that this can cause an immune response that cross-reacts with the gluten and the neurons, causing subclinical brain inflammation resulting in age-related dementia. Dr. Hyman recommends a gluten-free diet for everyone to prevent this detrimental pro-inflammatory response in the brain.

What makes these young cereal grasses so important is their outstanding nutrient profile. The most nutritious part of these plants resides in their young green blades of grass, which provide great health and antiaging benefits. These delicate grasses are highly perishable, and prior to modern-day processing techniques, were not widely available. Fortunately, we can now capture and protect the abundant nutrients of freshly harvested young green cereal grasses, the result of decades of research by the renowned scientist and physician Yoshihide Hagiwara, M.D. And though there are numerous brands of green foods on the natural food markets' shelves, only one contains the active living essence of the young barley grass plant, and that is Green Magma.

After researching more than two hundred types of edible vegetables and green plant leaves, Dr. Hagiwara determined that the concentrated green juice of young barley grass contained a perfect balance of beneficial phytonutrients. Using his years of experience in the pharmaceutical industry and performing pharmaceutical research, Dr. Hagiwara developed an award-winning juice extraction and spray-drying process to concentrate all the nutrients from barley grass juice into a convenient-to-use dry powder known today as Green Magma. He went on to develop a number of other whole food supplements using barley grass juice and other nutritious plant substances.

With his colleagues and staff at his plant headquarters in Oita, Japan, Dr. Hagiwara isolated and investigated the properties of barley grass and various plant foods. He and his fellow researchers at his Japan Pharmaceutical Development Company, along with leading researchers at Japanese universities, the University of California at Davis, and George Washington University, have investigated the many health benefits of barley grass juice, including its actions related to controlling cholesterol levels, increasing energy levels, modulating inflammation, antioxidation, detoxification, hormonal control, cardiovascular support, and immunity. Japan Pharmaceutical, the company that Dr. Hagiwara founded, continues his legacy of scientific inquiry at its research and development laboratory in Japan and in collaboration with scientists at leading institutions worldwide to further knowledge of the health benefits of barley grass juice and other plants.

It was initial studies demonstrating Green Magma's proven ability to decrease inflammation that first drew my attention. As I continued my own research in conjunction with enjoying liberal amounts of Green Magma daily, I recognized that its health benefits were numerous, especially for my women patients.

Antioxidant Protection

Green Magma provides key nutrition for women of all ages, especially during both menopause and postmenopause, when nutrient status becomes particularly critical. Green Magma contains flavonoids, but, unlike those found in soy, they are not isoflavones and don't act as phytoestrogens. Two major flavonoids in barley grass, saponarin and lutonarin, are potent antioxidants. Green Magma also contains the antioxidants alpha-carotene, beta-carotene, vitamin C, vitamin E succinate, superoxide dismutase (SOD), catalase, and chlorophyll. This synergistic array of antioxidants includes both water-soluble and fat-soluble types, ensuring that all of the body's cells are protected against oxidation within their cellular matrix and at their outer membrane surface. Women's antioxidant levels decrease during menopause. By increasing the intake of antioxidants through diet and supplements, menopausal symptoms and postmenopausal health concerns related to antioxidant status may be offset. These include cardiovascular disease—the number one cause of death in women—and disorders of the skeletal systems.

Cardiovascular Protection

During menopause, a decrease in the body's levels of antioxidants, including vitamin C, vitamin E, glutathione, and superoxide dismutase, among others, is accompanied by an increase in oxidative stress. Increased levels of oxidized cholesterol rather than cholesterol levels alone in the body are associated with an increased risk of coronary artery disease. A diet rich in fruits, vegetables, and whole food supplements like Green Magma containing a variety of antioxidants including SOD, as well as supplements of alpha-lipoic acid, Co Q10, omega-3s, vitamin C, astaxanthin, carnitine, and vitamin E, may help improve a woman's total antioxidant status during menopause, providing protection against excessive oxidative stress, and supporting healthy cardiovascular function. Clinical research has shown that Green Magma may directly address cardiovascular health concerns, since it lowers the level of markers of oxidative stress in the blood and inhibits the oxidation of low-density lipoprotein (LDL), while increasing serum levels of the antioxidant vitamins C and E.

Bone Support

In chapter 5 we will learn about the critical importance of healthy bones. As women age and approach menopause, declining estrogen levels can take their toll. Although the precise mechanisms whereby estrogen prevents bone loss have not yet been fully elucidated, there is evidence to suggest that the bone-sparing effects of estrogen may be mediated through antioxidants and that antioxidants may also help offset estrogen-deficient bone loss during menopause. Oxygen free radicals stimulate osteoclasts, the cells that resorb or break down bone. In animals, bone loss results from the removal of estrogen by removing the ovaries, and the administration of antioxidants has been shown to prevent ovariectomy-induced bone loss.

A recent in vitro study suggests that osteoclasts, the cells responsible for bone resorption, increase their activity in response to elevated levels of inflammatory cytokines as a result of increased oxidative stress. The presence of estrogen, however, stimulates the osteoclasts to increase production of the antioxidant glutathione peroxidase, which degrades the free-radical hydrogen peroxide into water and oxygen, rendering it harmless. Ovariectomized animals show increased bone resorption, which is prevented by the administration of either estrogen or catalase. The latter is an endogenous enzyme that, like glutathione peroxidase, breaks down hydrogen peroxide into water and oxygen. Thus, catalase prevents ovariectomy-induced bone loss. Researchers in a 2005 study at St. George's Hospital Medical School in the UK published "Hydrogen Peroxide Is Essential for Estrogen-Deficiency Bone Loss and Osteoclast Formation," in which they concluded that "hydrogen peroxide is the reactive oxygen species responsible for signaling the bone loss of estrogen deficiency."

Other studies have found that vitamin C or the carotenoid antioxidants may help prevent bone loss during menopause, although these were both preliminary findings and additional studies are needed to confirm this effect. Since there is a dramatic decrease in the production of estrogen by the ovaries during menopause along with an accelerated increase in bone resorption by the body, followed by a period of more gradual bone loss during the postmenopausal years, it would seem advisable to increase the intake of antioxidant-rich foods and supplements during menopause. Increasing the levels of intracellular antioxidants in women during menopause and the postmenopausal years may help decrease bone resorption by neutralizing hydrogen peroxide.

The barley grass in Green Magma has been shown to contain a high level of antioxidants, including catalase and carotenoids, along with many other nutrients to help the body increase in overall antioxidant status, and therefore may be useful in supporting normal bone mass during menopause and beyond. Of course, in order for antioxidants to help prevent bone resorption, the intake of adequate amounts of minerals, including calcium, magnesium, boron, silica, and omega-3s, as well as vitamins D and K2, is also needed—more about this in chapter 5. **I repeat: green foods are rich sources of bioavailable minerals that play a role in the prevention of bone resorption and in stimulating healthy bone remineralization.**

In addition to antioxidants, Green Magma and other green-food supplements by Green Foods Corporation are good sources of vitamin K. As we saw in chapter 3, vitamin K is important for both blood clotting and bone formation through its action as a cofactor in the carboxylation of certain proteins. In a well-known study that followed more than 72,000 women for ten years, researchers found that women with the lowest intake of vitamin K had a 30 percent higher risk of hip fracture than women with the highest intake of vitamin K. Although some studies have not found a direct link between bone mineral density and vitamin K intake, there is sufficient evidence to suggest that adequate amounts of vitamin K are necessary for bone health. A vegetable-rich diet supplies other nutrients important for bone building as well as vitamin K2, vitamin D, calcium, and the other minerals discussed in chapter 5. Taking Green Magma and other whole green-food supplements may help ensure adequate amounts of bone-building nutrients, especially for women during menopause and beyond.

Aging Gracefully with Astaxanthin

As you know, the brilliant, vibrant kaleidoscope of colors found in fruits, vegetables, beans, and legumes, as well as in nuts, extra-virgin olive oil, and seafood such as wild salmon signifies the presence of antioxidants in foods, making these foods an essential part of the Forever Young program. The carotenoid family of antioxidants offers very special and targeted properties for cellular rejuvenation for many reasons, not the least of which is their role in cellular growth and repair.

I am one of wild salmon's most vocal and enthusiastic proponents. There are many reasons for this, including the outstanding quality of its protein, so critical to cellular repair; its rich component of anti-inflammatory omega-3 essential fatty acids, essential for heart, skin, and brain health; and the presence of high levels of the carotenoid astaxanthin, which has myriad benefits, including superior anti-inflammatory properties. I recently met with the leading scientists at Fuji Health Science, a division of Fuji Chemical, global leaders in the production of astaxanthin. They generously shared with me the latest news and research on this remarkable carotenoid.

The King of Carotenoids

Astaxanthin is one of the most powerful all-natural antioxidants known to science and an irreplaceable key to any successful antiaging regimen. Often referred to as the "king of carotenoids," astaxanthin provides the greatest protection against damage to our bodies by reactive oxygen species such as singlet oxygen, which can result in lipid peroxidation (oxidation of fat). As we will learn in this chapter, astaxanthin is the key to mitigating the damaging effects of these oxidative assailants in every cell of our body.

What Is Astaxanthin?

Astaxanthin, a member of the carotenoid family of natural pigments, is closely related to beta-carotene, zeaxanthin, and lutein. This powerful, natural, biological antioxidant is found most abundantly in seafood. It gives the pink and red color to salmon, shrimp, and lobster. Since we cannot produce astaxanthin ourselves, we have to depend on our diet to obtain it as well as other carotenoids.

Let's take the case of salmon to demonstrate evolution at work. For salmon, the antioxidant power of astaxanthin is indispensable. Having evolved with a unique life cycle that demands more physical exertion than any other fish, salmon require protection against the damaging effects of reactive oxygen species (ROS) or free radicals, especially singlet oxygen, the most damaging of the ROS, generated during the rigorous journey from the sea back up the rivers and rapids to spawn. Salmon store the astaxanthin in their bodies, and it produces the deep orange, pink, or red color of their flesh as they grow and mature in the ocean, preparing for their final life cycle journey up the river to spawn.

Where Is Astaxanthin Found?

The most abundant source of astaxanthin in nature is the single-cell microalga *Haematococcus pluvialis*, which accumulates astaxanthin in lipid (fat) vesicles (small, anatomically normal sac- or bladderlike structures) during periods of nutrient deficiency and environmental stress. Since *H. pluvialis* often grows in places that are exposed to intense sunlight, during its dormant phase astaxanthin functions to protect the cell nucleus against free radicals generated by ultraviolet (UV) radiation, thus preventing damage to its DNA and preventing lipid peroxidation.

Astaxanthin serves the same purpose for all life forms as it moves up the food chain from a single-celled microalga to krill to salmon to human. This purpose is protection against oxidative damage, whether caused by UV radiation, excess physical exertion, or diabetes-generated glucose toxicity, or by many other sources of oxidative stress.

This astaxanthin-producing microalga is naturally found in arctic marine environments as well as freshwater rock pools all over the world. These are great sources of astaxanthin for aquatic life, flamingos, whose brilliant plumage is also the result of their astaxanthin-rich diet, and other animals, but they are not practical sources of astaxanthin for humans. Fortunately, there is an answer to this challenge. Cultivation facilities have been developed throughout the world to grow this astaxanthin-producing microalga. A leading cultivation technology developed by the Japanese pharmaceutical company Fuji Chemical Industry employs the concept of fully enclosed biosystems designed for maximum control and purity. The trade name of Fuji's premium all-natural astaxanthin is AstaREAL.

Unlocking the Secrets of Astaxanthin

Astaxanthin actually does only one thing well—but that one thing has an impact on all the cells in our body, including all the cells in our organ systems: it provides us with a highly effective defense against oxidative stress, which has a direct impact on damaging cellular inflammation and the inflammatory process.

Here is a brief summary of the benefits of the king of carotenoids.

ANTIOXIDANT CAPACITY   Astaxanthin is a lipid-soluble (fat-soluble) antioxidant that has been shown to provide exceptional protection against lipid peroxidation at the cellular level. Astaxanthin is also a powerful free-radical fighter. As you know, oxygen is a two-edged sword; it sustains life because it is essential for energy production in the mitochondria, but it becomes dangerous when it loses an electron and becomes a free radical, or reactive oxygen species. Astaxanthin has the ability to scavenge singlet oxygen, which is a damaging reactive oxygen species (ROS). However, to put astaxanthin's superior power into perspective, three separate studies comparing astaxanthin with other well-known antioxidants demonstrated astaxanthin to be 1,000 times more effective than vitamin E (alpha-tocopherol) against lipid oxidation and 550 times more effective against singlet oxygen.

CELL MEMBRANE POSITIONING   Astaxanthin has a unique structure. It is a lipid-soluble polyene chain with a polar region at either end. This structure allows astaxanthin to penetrate the bilayer of the cell membrane, protecting both the lipid center layer and the water-loving outer layers. When the cells undergo oxidative stress, transcription factors are activated, including NF-κB, which migrates to the nucleus and attaches to the DNA, resulting in cellular production of pro-inflammatory cytokines—the so-called serial killers of the cellular world. This ability to protect the cell membrane against oxidative attack is the key to suppressing the activation of NF-κB, which is the signaling compound responsible for the initiation of inflammation.

ANTI-INFLAMMATORY EFFECT   Several studies have shown the ability of astaxanthin to reduce inflammation, which could be considered the underlying mechanism for its many beneficial effects. In one study, it was shown to play a role in cytokine regulation by inhibiting the expression of inflammatory cytokines and chemokines.

Aging Gracefully

Astaxanthin is the underlying defender of your body, helping to protect and amplify the defense of your cells. It is involved with the major systems of the body, including the skin, the largest organ in the body; the cardiovascular system; and the muscles, the source of your vitality.

Skin Health, Age, and Beauty

Regardless of age, most women perceive wrinkles as heralding the loss of the skin's youth and beauty.

Skin is composed of three layers: the epidermis, the dermis, and the subcutaneous fat layer. The dermis contains collagen, elastin, and other fibers that support the skin's structure. These elements give skin a smooth, youthful appearance. The dermis, our "outer defense" layer, is the part of the skin most readily damaged by UV radiation. As you will learn, taking astaxanthin supplements is of critical importance in keeping the skin youthful and supple.

Antiwrinkle Mechanism

The UV radiation that affects the skin is composed of two types of waves, UVA and UVB. UVB rays are shorter than UVA rays and are the main cause of melanin production. However, it is the UVA rays, with their longer wavelength, that are responsible for much of the damage associated with photoaging. UVA rays penetrate deep into the dermis, where they damage collagen fibers, leading to wrinkle formation (Figure 1).

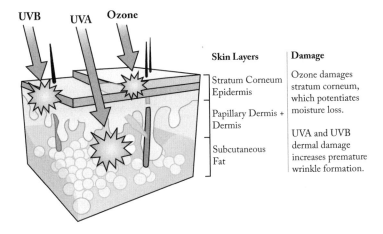

Skin Layers	Damage
Stratum Corneum Epidermis	Ozone damages stratum corneum, which potentiates moisture loss.
Papillary Dermis + Dermis	
Subcutaneous Fat	UVA and UVB dermal damage increases premature wrinkle formation.

FIGURE 1   The effects of UVA, UVB, and ozone on the skin.

UV rays induce the production of radical oxygen species (ROSs) and matrix metalloproteinases (MMPs) within the cells of the body exposed to the UV rays. These factors are the root of wrinkle formation because they destroy the collagen matrix in the dermis. Something discussed in chapter 2 bears repeating here. You have heard endlessly that excess exposure to UV radiation is hugely damaging to the skin. UV radiation increases free-radical activity in the cell plasma membrane, which releases arachidonic acid, the precursor of numerous pro-inflammatory chemicals including the prostaglandins and HETEs. This activates transcription factors such as NF-κB and AP-1. These in turn upregulate negative genes that produce pro-inflammatory cytokines that damage skin cells. When transcription factors such as AP-1 are activated, they produce and release collagen-digesting proteins (matrix metalloproteinase), resulting in microscarring in the deep portion of the skin called the dermis. The multiple *micro*scars lead to *macro*scarring, and this is how wrinkles are born.

The skin's repair mechanism will rebuild the damaged collagen but can be compromised by repeated exposure to uncontrolled levels of ROS and MMP, which then leads to the formation of wrinkles. The

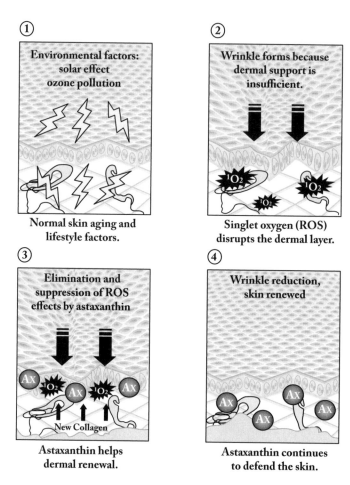

FIGURE 2   Astaxanthin supports skin renewal by attenuating factors that contribute to wrinkle formation.

presence of astaxanthin attenuates the effects of reactive oxygen and MMP, allowing the skin to regenerate properly (Figure 2). This leads to an improvement in the appearance of wrinkles as well as the texture and complexion of the skin.

Human clinical studies conducted with AstaREAL astaxanthin and performed in Japan and the United States showed significant improvement in the appearance of wrinkles as well as the elasticity and moisture content of the skin after only four weeks of supplementation.

Vitality:
The Ageless Quality of Life

When considering the concept of antiaging, we usually think in terms of longevity, which is something most of us would like to improve. Regardless of the number of years we may live, we would like those years to provide us with the highest quality of life possible. This is something that astaxanthin can play a key role in achieving.

Astaxanthin's significant anti-inflammatory power is vital to the maintenance of youthful vitality. At the heart of what ails us as we age is that insidious inflammatory process. Whether it affects our cardiovascular system or our joints, inflammation can and will rob us of the zest for life. The first benefit we will focus on in this section is how astaxanthin can help us maintain cardiovascular health.

Boosting Cardiovascular Health with Astaxanthin

The cardiovascular system is obviously critical to the health and vitality of us all, especially as we age. Elevated blood pressure is usually the first sign of developing trouble in our cardiovascular system. If there was a way to help maintain cardio health and normal blood pressure without extreme or artificial intervention, how welcome it would be. Astaxanthin has shown an indication that it can help do just that. In a recent study performed on postmenopausal women, a significant reduction in both systolic and diastolic blood pressure was shown after eight weeks of AstaREAL astaxanthin supplementation. Supporting this finding, four earlier laboratory studies, one performed in the United States and three in Japan, showed a significant reduction in blood pressure following supplementation with astaxanthin in controlled animal subjects.

Another consideration as we age is blood flow, especially peripheral capillary blood flow. As the circulation in our legs begins to decrease, unwanted symptoms begin to occur. Two separate studies validate astaxanthin's ability to improve blood flow. First, in a human blood rheology study, astaxanthin supplementation created significant improvement in capillary blood flow. To further support this suggested benefit, a study with astaxanthin supplementation was done that showed a significant increase in ankle brachial pressure index (ABI), suggesting reduced lower limb vascular resistance—in simpler terms, better blood flow in our legs.

At the heart of astaxanthin's support to the cardiovascular system is its ability to protect the body from lipid peroxidation. This ability of astaxanthin helps prevent the oxidation of LDL cholesterol, which is the key to maintaining a healthier blood lipid environment, thereby reducing the tendency for plaque buildup in the arteries. In another recent human study, astaxanthin supplementation showed a significant decrease in blood serum triglyceride and an increase in HDL cholesterol levels. A number of recent studies have shown that when this ratio is lowered, the risk of cardiovascular events is reduced.

Triathletes, Take Your Cue from Salmon!

Another outstanding benefit of astaxanthin relating to our vitality is its ability to increase muscle endurance and recovery. The amazing physical endurance salmon demonstrate on their arduous journey up the rapids and rivers to their spawning grounds led to the investigation of astaxanthin as related to physical endurance in humans. A number of animal and human studies have shown that astaxanthin can increase and improve muscle endurance as well as reduce muscle damage.

All physical activity, whether at work, sport, or leisure, generates reactive oxygen species (ROSs), and the more intense the activity, the greater the number of free radicals produced. **For years I have been telling my patients that I do not recommend vigorous activity for more than forty-five minutes, because the free radicals generated overwhelm our endogenous antioxidant protective mechanisms, with re-**

sulting negative effects on our overall health and fitness. Once again, moderation is the key.

ROSs have been shown to have damaging effects on muscle performance and recovery. The mitochondria are important to physical activity and are often referred to as the powerhouse of the cell, providing as much as 95 percent of our body's energy, primarily by the burning of muscle glycogen and fatty acids. A portion of this energy produces highly reactive and damaging ROSs, which in turn cause damage to the cell membrane and DNA. In addition, ROSs, activate the inflammatory response whereby monocytes migrate into the muscle tissue, causing additional cell damage. The resulting symptoms of muscle damage are tiredness and soreness. These symptoms can be brought on by any physical activity from a strenuous sport to daily household chores and at any stage in our lives, but the effects are more pronounced as we age. Astaxanthin has demonstrated three important physical benefits in clinical trials and supporting studies:

- Increased endurance
- Reduced muscle damage
- Improved lipid metabolism (fat burning)

One of several human clinical trials demonstrating astaxanthin's ability to improve endurance was performed in 1998 by a Swedish team of researchers. They conducted a randomized, double-blind, placebo-controlled study in which healthy male students were separated into an astaxanthin supplementation group and a placebo group. Each group was measured for endurance by performing squats with a 97-pound barbell at the start of the study and after three and six months. After six months, the subjects taking astaxanthin performed significantly more squats than the subjects taking the placebo, an increase of 56 percent.

One study demonstrating the protective effect of astaxanthin against muscle damage was performed in Japan in an animal model. Analysis of the muscles was performed in both the astaxanthin and the placebo groups following intense physical activity. The astaxanthin group showed significantly lower peroxidation damage. Other biochemical markers for oxidative damage and inflammation, such as DNA, creatine kinase (also known as creatine phosphokinase), and myeloperoxidase activity, were also significantly reduced in the astaxanthin-treated exercise group. These effects indicate that astaxanthin has a role in helping to protect muscle cell components and downregulating the inflammatory process.

Finally, a study was recently performed demonstrating that the astaxanthin-supplemented group had increased lipid metabolism rather than carbohydrate metabolism as the main source of energy during strenuous activity. This is a dream come true—burning fat instead of carbs! These methods of action are similar to the omega-3s aiding in the burning of fats and the partitioning of energy away from fat storage as described on page 79. I recommend that you take omega-3s along with your astaxanthin supplements for this synergistic action. In addition, analysis of the mitochondrial lipid transport enzyme known as carnitine palmitoyltransferase 1 (CPT1) revealed increased fat transferred into the mitochondria to be utilized more efficiently for energy and reduced oxidative damage in the presence of astaxanthin. This process not only has the effect of sustaining the energy output of muscle cells but also has a potential for the improvement of body composition and fat placement.

You do not need to be a world-class athlete to benefit from the effect of astaxanthin on muscle endurance. We can all use a bit more stamina, regardless of age or vocation. Remember: as we age, we gradually lose muscle mass, which weakens our bodies and makes us more prone to falls and injuries as well as age-related illnesses exacerbated by inactivity. Keeping your muscles strong and healthy will sustain the quality of your life.

Summary: Astaxanthin

Astaxanthin is a natural antioxidant with exceptional capacity that far exceeds that of most other antioxidant compounds. It has been shown to have nutritional and antiaging benefits that best fit the needs of the active and vital lifestyle of both the young and the aging.

When considering supplementation with astaxanthin, it is important to put your trust in a material that is not only supported by research but also produced in state-of-the-art facilities with the highest standards of product purity. This is why I recommend and support the one source of astaxanthin that fits both of these criteria: the AstaREAL brand astaxanthin produced by Fuji Chemical Industry Company in fully enclosed systems in Hawaii and Sweden. Fuji has also sponsored more than forty clinical studies to establish the health benefits of astaxanthin as well as more than thirty safety studies to provide its reliability. AstaREAL is also the brand of astaxanthin that attained GRAS (generally recognized as safe) status in January 2010 following an FDA review of Fuji's GRAS application. GRAS status also allows AstaREAL astaxanthin to be used as an ingredient in food and beverages.

24-Carrot Gold

No discussion of foods that renew, repair, and rejuvenate would be complete without the most significant sources of the carotenoids, both those found in microalgae and fish such as salmon (astaxanthin) and those found in plants (lycopene, lutein, zeaxanthin, alpha-carotene, and beta-carotene). The brilliant colors of the plants, fish, and fowl are the result of these natural antioxidant pigments and impart eye appeal and serious eye protection and regeneration. Green Foods doesn't just specialize in greens, although that is a big part of its expertise. Dr. Hagiwara also did extensive work with a wide variety of vegetables, including carrots—aptly named due to their rich complement of (no surprise) carotenoids.

Carrot Essence is an excellent source of two of nature's most powerful antioxidants: carotenoids (including alpha-carotene and beta-carotene) and vitamin C, combined in a delicious whole-food beverage powder. As we saw in the astaxanthin section of this chapter, carotenoids are vital to cellular growth and repair.

The fresh organic carrots are harvested at their nutritional peak, washed, juiced, and then spray-dried in a temperature-controlled manner to stabilize their nutrients. Organic maltodextrin, a complex carbohydrate, is added to coat the delicate nutrients and protect them from harmful oxidation. Carrot Essence also contains acerola powder, a potent natural source of vitamin C made from the acerola berry. Carrot Essence contains no added sugar, salt, colorings, or fillers and is free of animal products, gluten, soy, wheat, and yeast. The finished product is in a fine powder form, easily mixed with beverages.

Carrot Essence contains more than 200 percent of the recommended daily amount (RDA) of vitamin A and 55 percent of the RDA of vitamin C in a single serving. After more than thirty years of scientific research, the medical community and nutrition experts agree that antioxidants, especially beta-carotene and vitamin C, play important roles in promoting health and longevity. Carrot Essence is supplied as a fraction of the whole food, an extremely important point, because taking isolated carotenoid supplements such as just beta-carotene proved, in a large study, to be detrimental! For example, in a study of smokers who were taking isolated beta-carotene supplements, the researchers noted a greater risk of lung cancer than in those not taking the isolated carotenoid. In this wonderful whole-food extract supplement, all of the carotenoids are present, avoiding the negative consequences of the isolated nutrient and giving us all of the expected benefits of the mixed carotenoids.

The Roles and Benefits of Carotenes in the Body

The carotenoids in Carrot Essence are precursors of vitamin A, which is crucial for maintaining healthy skin, eyesight, mucous membranes, immunity, liver function, teeth, and bones. Unlike vitamin A, however, alpha- and beta-carotene are nontoxic at sustained high levels, since the body makes only the amount of vitamin A it needs from them. When there is sufficient vitamin A in the body, the conversion of alpha-carotene and beta-carotene to vitamin A ceases.

Cell-to-Cell Communication

The carotene molecules that are not converted into vitamin A are powerful antioxidants that neutralize free radicals before these radicals can cause serious damage to our tissues. Beta-carotene is normally present in high concentrations in the blood and is naturally incorporated into low-density lipoprotein (LDL) molecules and serves to inhibit the oxidation of LDL, thereby lowering the risk of type 2 diabetes and cardiovascular disease. In addition, the established ability of beta-carotene to both inhibit lipid peroxidation and promote cellular communication may endow this carotene with anticarcinogenic properties. Studies indicate that this cell-to-cell communication is important in preventing cancer by increasing the activity of a molecule called Connexin 43. This molecule forms small channels between cells, connecting virtually all the cells in the body. Through these channels, cells exchange nutrients and vital signals that ensure normal cellular growth.

One of the reasons that carotenoids are so vital to cellular health is the fact that they are fat-soluble, which enables them to enter both the cell plasma membrane and the mitochondria. They are able to protect these parts of the cell from oxidative stress, free-radical damage, and pro-inflammatory chemicals. This capability provides exceptional protection to our immune system, critically important in this era of potential pandemics. It is well known that our immune cells are especially sensitive to oxidative stress.

Low beta-carotene levels are associated with the decline in cognitive function in those with Alzheimer's disease, so adequate levels of beta-carotene, as well as other carotenoids, may help protect against the development of this disease and promote healthy brain function throughout life. The presence of the carotenoid astaxanthin in wild salmon might be another reason why fish has long been considered "brain food."

Here are some of the key benefits you may enjoy from eating carotenoid-rich foods:

- The body converts the carotenoids in carrots, spinach, and other vegetables to vitamin A (retinol) as needed.
- Carotenoids may reduce the risk of cardiovascular disease, in part because of their antioxidant, anti-inflammatory properties. (Unlike food sources, supplemental carotenoids such as alpha- and beta-carotene do not produce consistently positive results against cardiovascular disease.)
- Carotenoids neutralize the free radicals responsible for general oxidative stress. The cellular damage and inflammation created by oxidative stress accelerates the internal aging process and manifests externally as wrinkles.
- Carotenoids offer protection from a number of cancers, including lung, bladder, breast, esophagus, and stomach.
- Carotenoids protect against wrinkles and skin cancer by helping to block sunlight-induced inflammation in the skin.
- The lutein and zeaxanthin abundant in spinach, kale, and collard greens exert protective antioxidant effects in the retina and thus appear to help prevent cataracts and macular degeneration. These foods also help prevent prostatic changes.

Synergy with Vitamin C

Vitamin C, a water-soluble vitamin, is located in many tissues, including blood vessels, and may be protective against the oxidation of LDL, since low vitamin C levels in the aorta have been found in people with cardiovascular disease. Together, beta-carotene and vitamin C may offer synergistic protection against cardiovascular disease. In addition, both of these antioxidants complement the actions of vitamin E in preventing oxidation of LDL and other biomolecules. Beta-carotene is a fat-soluble antioxidant while vitamin C is a water-soluble antioxidant, and together they provide antioxidant protection to both the lipid and the aqueous portions of our body's cellular matrix.

The Importance of Whole-Food Antioxidants

Carrot Essence is made from fresh-squeezed organic carrot juice and whole acerola berries and contains all the nutrients, cofactors, and diverse antioxidants found naturally in these two whole foods. Observational studies show that people with the highest levels of carotenoids in their diets have a reduced risk of several chronic diseases. As mentioned, intervention trials of beta-carotene supplements indicate that this supplement taken alone may be of little value in preventing cardiovascular disease and cancer in well-nourished individuals. Taking the isolated nutrients is counterproductive, and the whole-food essence is recommended.

Since total antioxidant capacity (TAC) is a predictor of plasma beta-carotene levels, the body's level of beta-carotene depends on the variety and amounts of other antioxidants present in the body. Obtaining antioxidants from whole-food sources helps ensure that we receive a greater diversity and level of antioxidant protection.

Antioxidants work in concert, acting synergistically, and the body requires a variety of both water-soluble and fat-soluble antioxidants for optimal protection against free radicals. Carrot Essence is a concentrated, bioavailable source of the potent antioxidants, carotenoids and vitamin C, conveniently provided in a whole-food form. Antioxidant protection of all the tissues in the body including the cardiovascular system helps ensure cellular nourishment and healthful longevity.

Omega-3 Essential Fatty Acids and Life Span: The Long and Short of It

Omega-3

As you will learn later in this chapter, stress plays a role in shortening life span, and I will retell several excellent news stories that Craig Weatherby and the team at Vital Choice generously shared with me. The good news is that certain nutrients, such as omega-3 essential fatty acids, can help counteract this effect. I have long championed the benefits of wild salmon and other cold-water fish for a variety of reasons, including their ability to keep skin supple, youthful, and radiant; increase brainpower and cardiovascular health; protect joints; and improve and stabilize mood, to name just a few benefits. I believe there is a solid link between diet and disease, including some forms of cancer. I also believe—and science bears this out—that stress is one of the single greatest precipitators of accelerated aging.

If we are to be Forever Young, we need to find successful strategies to conquer stress, both physical and mental. A loving, nonjudgmental companion animal is a great antidote to stress, as are forms of exercise such as yoga (see chapter 7), spending time out in nature, or simply making the time to restore yourself.

Stress can shorten your life span—this is not a theory but an actual measurable fact. A recent study at the University of California has not only implicated stress in cell aging, it also suggests that stress accelerates the rate at which cells age. We have long known that stress precipitates premature aging, but the exact mechanism of how this occurs has been unclear.

According to researchers, stress affects telomeres, strips of DNA at the end of chromosomes, which appear to protect and stabilize the chromosome ends. A chromosome is a type of cell that carries hereditary information. Telomeres are involved in regulating cell division. Each time the cell divides, the telomere shortens, until eventually there is nothing left, making cell division less reliable and increasing the risk of age-related disorders. Like the wrapped tips of shoelaces, without which the laces would unravel, telomeres ensure that a cell's chromosomes do not fuse with one another or rearrange themselves during cell division, which can lead to cancer.

With each replication the telomeres shorten, and when the telomeres are gone, the cells are programmed to commit a form of cellular "suicide" called apoptosis, which was discussed in chapter 1. Telomeres are highly vulnerable to oxidative stress from free radicals generated by:

- Eating a pro-inflammatory diet (i.e., high-glycemic carbohydrates)
- Environmental stressors
- Weakened immune system
- Excess exposure to ultraviolet light
- Hormonal changes
- Stress
- Normal metabolism

Since they protect telomeres by neutralizing free radicals, foods rich in antioxidants, which help the body neutralize free radicals, help maintain good health and a youthful appearance.

Omega-3s to the Rescue

Researchers have shown that omega-3s may also protect telomeres, as one study with heart patients demonstrates.

Researchers based at the University of California conducted a study designed to determine whether omega-3 blood levels were associated with changes in telomere length among heart patients with coronary artery disease.

> A team led by Ramin Farzaneh-Far, M.D., recruited 608 heart patients between September 2000 and December 2002 and measured the length of their leukocyte telomeres at the beginning of the study and again after five years of follow-up.
>
> After comparing the starting lengths of the cardiac out-patients' telomeres with their length after five years, the re-searchers found that people with the lowest omega-3 levels experienced the speediest rate of telomere shortening.
>
> In contrast, those with the highest omega-3 levels showed the slowest rate of telomere shortening.
>
> RESULTS MAY HELP EXPLAIN OMEGA-3s'
> PROVEN HEART BENEFITS
>
> The findings offer one plausible biological explanation for why eating cold-water fish such as salmon, sardines, and an-chovies as well as taking fish oil helps heart patients.
>
> The authors speculated that omega-3s may counteract oxidative stress, or increase the production of telomerase, an enzyme that lengthens and repairs shortened telomeres.
>
> If you find it surprising that they'd suggest an antioxi-dant role for omega-3s, you've been listening to the wrong people.

Many observers make erroneous assumptions about the susceptibility of dietary omega-3s to oxidation in the body.

While omega-3s oxidize rapidly when exposed to air, several recent studies have shown that they act as antioxidants inside our vascular system . . . thereby reducing inflammation and, in turn, the risk of atherosclerosis and cardiovascular disease. . . .

The researchers studied only the effects of fish oil on cellular aging in heart patients, so it is not clear if the association would hold true in healthy people.

But as Dr. Farzaneh-Far told Reuters, "There is no reason to think that it wouldn't."

He expressed the essence of his team's finding this way:

"Telomere length is an emerging marker for determining biological age. . . . We are excited to identify omega-3 fatty acids as a potentially protective factor that may slow down telomere shortening."

Mushroom Wisdom:
The Key to Preserving Youth, Beauty, Health, and Longevity

Throughout Asia, certain mushrooms have played important roles in maintaining health, preserving youth, and increasing longevity. Here is a description of the health benefits of seven long-studied medicinal mushrooms. With the exception of maitake, this is the first time that I have introduced these ancient and miraculous mushrooms to readers. This is a fertile area for further research to support the efficacy of ancient Eastern medications.

It has been both an honor and a tremendous learning experience to meet with Mike Shirota, one of the founders of Mushroom Wisdom, who introduced the finest-quality medicinal mushrooms to the U.S. market, and his team, including Shuji Matsubara and Donna Noonan, who have been so helpful in sharing scientific information included here. I first learned about maitake from Harry Preuss, MD, MACN, CNS, a physician and scientist at Georgetown University School of Medicine, who has undertaken a number of scientific studies on maitake for the company—with incredibly inspiring results.

Here is a short description of the outstanding healing and rejuvenating properties, background information on, and constituents of this remarkable group of mushrooms, all of which are available on MushroomWisdom.com.

Lion's Mane (*Hericium erinaceus*): The Brain Tonic

Lion's mane is a type of mushroom that has been used traditionally in China and Japan for hundreds of years and is also known as bear's head or monkey's head. The common name in English is hedgehog fungus and in Chinese is *hou tou gu*. This mushroom's most promising (and surprising) benefits include the ability to stimulate the synthesis of nerve growth factor, which may help inhibit brain dysfunction associated with Alzheimer's disease and other neurological diseases. Studies also confirm many of its traditional uses, such as supporting the digestive system and acting as a tonic for the nervous system.

Bioactivities

ANTI-COGNITIVE DECLINE   Stimulating activity of the synthesis of nerve growth factor (NGF), preventing and ameliorating senile dementia

ANTITUMOR   Immune enhancement, cytotoxic effect

DIGESTIVE TONIC   Treatment of stomach and duodenal ulcer and chronic atrophic gastritis; improvement of indigestion

Reishi (*Ganoderma lucidum*): The Longevity Mushroom

Reishi, which is called *ling zhi* in Chinese, *mannentake* or *reishi* in Japanese, and *young zhi* in Korean, is one of the most famous medicinal mushrooms in the world. It has been used as the "mushroom of immortality" for thousands of years. During the last two decades, researchers have found various bioactive constituents that have a wide range of actions, including boosting immune function, specifically natural killer cells, macrophage, and interferon, as well as antiviral and antibacterial functions; cardiovascular support; lowering blood pressure and serum cholesterol; and protecting the heart. Research has also demonstrated reishi's possible usefulness for allergies, bronchitis, cancer, HIV, inflammation, liver, and protection against radiation.

Bioactivities

ANTITUMOR Immune enhancement; increasing IL-2, IL-6, and TNF-α production; interferon-inducing activity; inducing cancer cell apoptosis; cytotoxic effect

ANTI-HIV Cytopathic effect; inhibiting HIV-1 PR enzyme

ANTIHYPERTENSION Inhibiting angiotensin-1-converting enzyme

ANTIDIABETES Enhances insulin sensitivity

ANTIHYPERLIPEMIA Inhibiting cholesterol biosynthesis, reduces triglycerides and LDL

HEPATOPROTECTION Lowering GOT and GPT; improving chronic hepatitis

ANTITHROMBOGENICITY Inhibiting platelet aggregation or formation of blood clots

ANTIALLERGY Inhibiting histamine release

CARDIOVASCULAR TONIC Increasing blood flow of coronary artery

Shiitake (*Lentinus edodes*):
Overall Energy and Liver Enhancer

Shiitake is the most popular edible mushroom in Asian cuisine, including the cuisines of China and Japan, and has been gaining popularity in the United States. This mushroom is so much more than just a delicious food. The pharmaceutical Lentinan is derived from shiitake and is one of three mushroom-based anticancer drugs approved by the Japanese Ministry of Health and Welfare in 1985. It exhibits strong immune responses and has been extensively studied for use with cancers and viral infections. Shiitake contains a variety of constituents that have demonstrated a wide range of actions, including immune modulation, antitumor, liver protection, cholesterol lowering, antiviral, and blood pressure–lowering. Its extract is also a potent antifungal agent, effective against *Candida albicans.*

Bioactivities

ANTITUMOR   Immune enhancement; activating macrophages, T cells, and NK cells, increasing production of TNF-α, interleukins, interferon, and complement C3

ANTI-HIV   Producing synergistic effect with azidothymidine (AZT)

ANTIHYPERLIPEMIA   Promoting the metabolism and excretion of ingested cholesterol

ANTITHROMBOGENICITY   Inhibiting platelet aggregation

NATURAL ANTIDOTE   Strengthening liver function; detoxication

Cordyceps (*Cordyceps sinensis*):
Stamina, Endurance, and Sex Drive

Cordyceps is called "winter worm, summer grass" in China and Japan because it is a fungus that "fruits" out of the head of dead worms or insects. While this may sound decidedly unappealing, cordyceps is a very rare and special mushroom—one that truly deserves its nickname "elixir of life."

Cordyceps can be found only at altitudes above 12,000 feet above sea level, in remote areas of southwest China and Nepal. Cordyceps is one of the most valuable and expensive herbs in traditional Chinese medicine. Historically, it was available only to the imperial family because of its great rarity and cost. In 1993, the women athletes of the Chinese national running team achieved nine world records at the World Track and Field Meet in Germany. One of them broke the record for the 10,000-meter run by an astounding forty-two seconds. What was their secret? The athletes gave credit to an intense training schedule and the use of cordyceps. Since then, this mushroom has received international attention, and its pharmacological properties have been evaluated in detail. It may be useful as an antiaging aid and in lowering high cholesterol, protecting the liver, increasing sex drive, and supporting cardiovascular health.

Bioactivities

CARDIOTONIC EFFECT   Strengthening the cardiac muscle

ENERGY ENHANCEMENT   Increasing erythrocytes, the relatively large red cells in the blood that transport oxygen from the lungs to all of the living tissue in the body; enhancing endurance

ANTIAGING   Preventing the formation of peroxide lipids; improving memory

ENHANCING SEX DRIVE AND ANTI-IMPOTENCE   Protecting the corpus cavernosum of the penis

HEPATOPROTECTION   Reducing the ascites seen in liver cirrhosis; prevents the formation of fibrosis and normalizes the liver enzymes SGOT and SGPT

KIDNEY TONIC   Ameliorating aminoglycoside nephrotoxicity

ANTITUMOR Enhancing depressed immune functions

ANTIDIABETES Increasing insulin secretion

ANTIHYPERTENSION Dilating coronary artery; increasing blood flow

STOMACH TONIC Inhibiting the formation of stress-related stomach ulcers

Royal Agaricus (*Agaricus blazei Murill*): Super Immune Booster

Originating in the mountain region of Piedade, Brazil, royal agaricus has gained popularity in its home country as well as in Asia as a panacea (cure-all). Royal agaricus is also used to treat cancer. Interest in this medicinal mushroom was first piqued when it was recognized that people living in this region had a significantly lower rate of disease, including lower cancer rates. Research done in Japan in the 1980s and 1990s supports these benefits. Studies have demonstrated the role of royal agaricus for use in the recovery from cancer and in lowering blood glucose and serum cholesterol levels and blood pressure. It is also known to possess strong immune enhancement properties. In Brazil, agaricus is called *cogumelo de Deus*, which translates as "mushroom of God."

Bioactivities

ANTITUMOR Immune enhancement; activating macrophages, T cells, and NK cells; increasing TNF-α production; inducing cancer cell apoptosis and cytotoxicity

ANTIHYPERLIPEMIA Lowering total cholesterol; increasing HDL cholesterol and lowering LDL cholesterol; preventing arteriosclerosis

IMPROVES HEPATITIS Lowering liver enzymes SGOT, SGPT, and GGTP, improving liver functions

ANTIALLERGY Immunoregulating effect

ANTIAGING   Eliminating free radicals; preventing the formation of peroxide lipids (oxidized fats); improving age-related disorders

Turkey Tail (*Coriolus versicolor*): Polysaccharide Power

Although this may be your first exposure to turkey tail, historically known in China as *yun zhi* and in Japan as *kawaratake*, it may just be the most studied medicinal mushroom of all. Polysaccharide kureha (PSK, also called krestin) was extracted from turkey tail in Japan in 1965 and polysaccharide peptide (PSP) in China in 1984. In Japanese trials, PSK significantly extended the survival rates of those with cancer of the stomach, colon-rectum, esophagus, nasopharynx, and lung. In 1977, PSK was the first polysaccharide antitumor drug derived from a mushroom to be approved by the Japanese Ministry of Health and Welfare for use as a cancer treatment. Not only did PSP show antitumor effects, but its significant antivirus and anti-inflammatory properties have proved effective in treating hepatitis B and chronic active hepatitis.

Bioactivities

ANTITUMOR   Immune enhancement, such as activating macrophages, T cells, and NK cells; enhancing serum C3 and IgG; promoting lymphocyte proliferation; increasing the production of interleukins and interferon

IMPROVES HEPATITIS   Lowering liver enzymes SGPT and SGOT; repairing damaged liver cells; normalizing liver function; minimizing the symptoms of hepatitis and cirrhosis

Tremella (*Tremella fuciformis*): Beautiful Skin, Strong Bones, Weight Control

Tremella, also known as "silver ear" or "white jerry leaf," is a very popular mushroom in Chinese cuisine. In traditional Chinese medicine, tremella extract is also used as a cough syrup for treating chronic tracheitis and other cough-related conditions such as asthma, dry cough, and heat in the lungs. It is said that Yang Guifei (719–756, an imperial concubine in the Tang dynasty), considered to be the greatest beauty in Chinese history, believed that the mushroom was critical in keeping her face and body youthful and beautiful. Tremella contains more than 70 percent dietary fiber such as acidic polysaccharides and is also very rich in vitamin D. Modern research has indicated its usefulness as an antitumor agent, for lowering blood glucose and cholesterol, and in protecting against radiation.

Bioactivities

HYPOCHOLESTEROLEMIC EFFECT   Inhibiting cholesterol absorption from the intestine; reducing cholesterol concentration in serum and liver; preventing arteriosclerosis

ANTIDIABETES   Improving the secretion of insulin by repairing damaged pancreatic beta-cells; promoting the absorption of glucose in the liver; inhibiting the release of glucose from the liver by increasing hexokinase activity; reducing glucose-6-phosphatase activity

ANTITUMOR   Immune enhancement, producing a synergistic effect by the combination of glucuronoxylomannan with mitomycin C

PREVENTION OF OSTEOPOROSIS   Enhancing calcium absorption

HEPATOPROTECTION   Promoting the metabolism of protein and nucleic acid in the liver

————

From cold-plasma technology and microcurrent to watercress and barley grass, from astaxanthin to ancient healing mushrooms, this chapter has provided you with a wide range of scientifically proven ways to slow down the clock, ward off disease, increase your vitality, and rejuvenate your body on a cellular level.

In the next chapter, we will further discuss the importance of bone health—how to achieve it and how to keep it, for a beautiful bone structure regardless of age.

Chapter Five

THE IMPORTANCE OF BONE HEALTH

When I started researching this chapter, I had no idea how radicalized I would become about healthy bones and their crucial function in all aspects of healthy aging and disease prevention. In fact, this is one of the most important chapters in this book because, as you will learn, healthy bones are the very foundation of our immune system, and until now, we did not have the most ideal strategies to ensure that we could prevent bone loss.

Bone formation—the acquisition of bone mineral density (BMD)—peaks between the ages of 20 and 30. **After the age of 35, both men and women begin to lose bone mass unless they take action to prevent it.** Unfortunately, at that age few of us are thinking about our health, our longevity, or anything in between. By the time we begin to think about our bones, we may have already suffered serious damage. It seems hard to believe that this can happen so early in our lives. Often our conception of age-related bone loss is that of a person of advanced age—seventies or eighties—bent under the burden of the dowager's hump.

You need to protect your bones from an early age. If you are in your twenties or thirties and reading this chapter, you can take active steps to prevent future problems. If you are older, take heart because there are exciting new strategies that can make a significant difference now.

Regular exercise is far and away the single most important action we can take to prevent and help reverse bone loss. Unfortunately, we are raising a generation of couch potatoes and computer/video jockeys who rarely exercise. If you happen to be a small Caucasian female with a penchant for dieting, the risk of bone loss is even greater. But there is good news. According to many studies, a high-intensity exercise program prevents bone loss in early postmenopausal women with low bone density.

The Weighting Game

As many studies affirm, weight-bearing exercises have an extremely beneficial effect on bone mass and bone density. The pressure exerted on the bones during this type of exercise stimulates the building of bone. Ideally, your exercise routines will be complex and will involve the total body; in this way you can achieve the greatest benefits. In chapter 7 you will find a comprehensive yoga program to increase physical and mental health and well-being—one designed to keep you Forever Young, or as close to it as reasonably possible.

A Step in the Right Direction

In conjunction with weight training, I recommend a thirty-minute brisk walk or jog every day. My colleague Harry Preuss, M.D., and I are firm believers in the use of pedometers to encourage an active lifestyle. A pedometer senses your body motion and counts your footsteps. If you are like me, you enjoy a challenge—and a pedometer motivates me to increase my movements. Many of us spend long hours in front of computers, and wearing the pedometer reminds us of just how sedentary our lives have become. If it is 10 A.M. and you glance at the pedometer and see that it is registering a meager 200 steps and your goal is 10,000 per day, it can help spur you into immediate action. I set a goal each day and am always delighted when I exceed it. **You need to take 6,000 steps per day for overall good health and as many as 10,000 steps per day for weight loss.** It is never too late to start an exercise program, and consistency is always the key. Walking is a great default exercise program in that you don't need a gym; the only equipment you need is a pair of good walking shoes, and, weather permitting, walking is something you can do 365 days a year.

Who Is at Risk?

According to information from the National Osteoporosis Foundation posted on the National Institute of Health's Web site (www.osteo.org), the following factors can put you at increased risk for osteoporosis:

- History of fracture after age 50.
- Current low bone mass.
- History of fracture in a close relative.
- Being female.
- Being thin and/or having a small frame.
- Advanced age (osteoporosis is a major public health threat for 55 percent of people 50 years of age and older; the older you are, the greater the risk).
- A family history of osteoporosis.
- Low lifetime calcium intake.
- Vitamin D deficiency.

- An inactive lifestyle.
- For women only: estrogen deficiency as a result of meno-pause, especially early or surgically induced. Also, women who stop menstruating before menopause because of conditions such as anorexia or bulimia or because of excessive physical exercise are at greater risk.
- For men only: low testosterone levels.
- For both men and women: use of certain medications to treat chronic medical conditions such as rheumatoid arthritis, endocrine disorders (i.e., an underactive thyroid, which can be helped by coconut oil), seizure disorders, and gastrointestinal diseases may have side effects that can damage bone and lead to osteoporosis. One class of drugs that has particularly damaging effects on the skeleton is gluco-corticoids (a group of steroids that have metabolic and anti-inflammatory effects). The following drugs can also cause bone loss:
  - Excessive thyroid hormones
  - Anticonvulsants
  - Antacids containing aluminum

These facts notwithstanding, the news is particularly grim for women. It is difficult to overstate the importance of BMD, which is often viewed as the "gold standard" for bone health. Unfortunately, for a variety of reasons, BMD is decreasing in women in the United States. In 2004, *Bone Health and Osteoporosis: A Report of the Surgeon General* predicted that by 2020 (a scant decade away) half of all American citizens older than 50 will be at risk for fractures from osteoporosis and low bone mass if no immediate action is taken. The report concluded that Americans' bone health is in jeopardy due to increasingly sedentary lifestyles, an absence of current information about bone health (which this chapter will hope to alleviate), and inadequate nutrition. The surgeon general recommended that people of all ages ensure that they get the recommended amounts of calcium and vitamin D, and that supplementation may be helpful. Pointing out that people are never too young or too old to improve their bone health, the surgeon general issued a "call to action" for the development and evaluation of bone health programs that incorporated three components: (1) improved health literacy, (2) increased physical activity, and (3) improved nutrition. Though this is a vitally important initiative for everyone, women in particular need to be educated on their risks, which pose a significant threat to BMD with the passing years.

Bone loss accelerates after menopause because the female hormone estrogen, needed to maintain bone density, is greatly reduced. The lack of estrogen accelerates a process known as *bone remodeling*, the process in which small areas of bone are destroyed and subsequently rebuilt. Estrogen deficiency can lead to an imbalance, resulting in more destruction and less formation, which can predispose women to osteoporosis as they age. If a woman's ovaries are surgically removed, even more rapid bone loss may occur because estrogen is made primarily in the ovaries. The most rapid rates of bone loss in women occur during the first five years after menopause, when the decrease in the production of estrogen results in increased bone resorption and decreased calcium absorption. In fact, according to statistics, women may lose as much as 3 to 5 percent of bone mass per year during the years immediately following menopause, with decreases of less than 1 percent per year after age 65. Two studies are in agreement that increased calcium intake during menopause *will not* completely offset menopause bone loss. Other studies show that nutritional supplements such as silicon in the form of choline-stabilized orthosilicic acid improves the bone health benefits of both calcium and vitamin D. As you will discover, specially targeted nutrients can not only slow bone loss, they can actually encourage new bone growth.

While there is an extensive and compelling body of research supporting the positive effects of calcium and vitamin D3 on bone health, a review of forty-eight studies on the effects of calcium on bone health concluded that other micronutrients are needed to optimize bone health, including vitamin K2, magnesium, and trace minerals. Vitamin C has also been reported as essential to collagen formation and normal bone development.

Healthy Bones, Healthy Heart

Vitamin K1

Many of us are familiar with vitamin K (phylloquinone, also known as phytonadione), commonly referred to as vitamin K1, which is a fat-soluble vitamin found in foods such as cabbage, broccoli, cauliflower, spinach, kale, turnip greens, and other dark leafy greens, cereals, and other vegetables. Vitamin K1 makes up about 90 percent of the vitamin K in a typical Western diet and plays an important role in blood clotting. Because this is a fat-soluble vitamin, it is important to eat these foods dressed with a little extra-virgin olive oil to ensure absorption of the nutrient. Some studies indicate that only 10 percent of the vitamin K1 in foods is absorbed by your body.

Today, emerging evidence in human intervention studies indicate that vitamin K1 at a much lower dose may also benefit bone health, in particular when coadministered with vitamin D. Several mechanisms are suggested by which vitamin K can modulate bone metabolism. Besides the gamma-carboxylation of osteocalcin, a protein believed to be involved in bone mineralization, there is increasing evidence that vitamin K positively affects calcium balance, a key mineral in bone metabolism. The Institute of Medicine has recently increased the dietary reference intakes of vitamin K to 90 micrograms per day for women and 120 micrograms per day for men, which is an increase of approximately 50 percent from previous recommendations.

A new analysis by Joyce McCann, Ph.D., and Bruce Ames, Ph.D., of Children's Hospital Oakland Research Institute of data from hundreds of published articles dating back to the 1970s also advises that the current recommendations for vitamin K intakes be increased.

Current recommendations are based on levels to ensure adequate blood coagulation, but failing to ensure long-term optimal levels of the vitamin may accelerate bone fragility, arterial and kidney calcification, cardiovascular disease, and possibly even cancer.

Vitamin K2: Don't Leave Home Without It!

Though this is good news, the news about vitamin K2 is even better when it comes to both bone and arterial health. Vitamin K2, also known as menaquinones, stays in the body for a significantly longer time than K1. It makes up about 10 percent of a typical Western diet's vitamin K and can be synthesized in the gut by microflora.

Menaquinones (MK-n) can also be found in the diet: MK-4 can be found in meat; MK-7, MK-8, and MK-9 are found in fermented food products like cheese, and an especially rich source of MK-7 is natto, a popular, centuries-old breakfast dish in Japan made from steamed fermented soybeans. Because of its rather unpleasant—some might call it "slimy"—consistency, natto, said to be the food of samurai warriors, can be a hard sell to the Western palate.

Chairman of the Board Certified

My friend and colleague Stephen Sinatra, M.D., F.A.C.N., C.N.S., is board certified in both internal medicine and cardiology. The buildup of arterial plaque is deadly to the healthy heart, and Dr. Sinatra continually searches for effective strategies to decrease this threat. A number of studies have demonstrated the effectiveness of vitamin K2 in reversing plaque in blood vessels. **Vitamin K2 appears to assist in the decalcification of hard plaque formations.**

Dr. Sinatra has seen outstanding progress in his patients taking the MK-7 (menaquinone-7) type of vitamin K2, which offers the following unique benefits:

- Provides the most active and bioavailable form of vitamin K2, MK-7
- Helps reduce the level of calcium in the bloodstream
- Supports cardiovascular health
- Helps strengthen bones
- Aids in calcium absorption by bones
- Helps increase bone density

I recently met with Dr. Sinatra to learn even more about this remarkable nutrient. Although this is a chapter on bone health, the remarkable discoveries about vitamin K2 demonstrate the holistic nature of the body and how all systems are intrinsically linked—in this instance, bone health and heart health. This makes it difficult to compartmentalize each organ system into a neat little chapter. There is tremendous overlap among bone health, digestive health, the immune system, the cardiovascular system, and so forth. As you will discover, a great bone structure means much more than just getting us on the pages of *Vogue*.

Dr. Sinatra had impressive news from Dr. Cees Vermeer, a biochemist from Maastricht University in the Netherlands and one of the top vitamin K2 researchers in the world. Two new studies (published in *Blood*, the journal of the American Society of Hematology) by Dr. Vermeer's team of researchers have reported the following:

The first study showed that vitamin K2 is more absorbable by the body than vitamin K1, so K2 is able to provide more support for the enzyme process that contributes to bone health—and more protection against osteoporosis. This absorbability puts vitamin K2 at greater risk of interfering with Coumadin, which is a vitamin K antagonist. Vitamin K promotes clotting, and Coumadin is prescribed to keep the blood thin by preventing clotting. According to Dr. Sinatra, new evidence from Europe suggests that Coumadin may also interfere with a vitamin K2 protein system that keeps calcium out of the arterial walls. It now appears that on one hand, Coumadin thins the blood, but on the other, it contributes to arterial calcification. Coumadin causes a deficiency of both vitamin K1 and vitamin K2. It should come as no surprise to learn that Coumadin takers suffer more osteoporosis in conjunction with more abnormal calcium deposits in other areas, such as the heart valves—in fact, twice as much as those not taking the drug. Dr. Sinatra has become extremely cautious about prescribing Coumadin because of these risks, reserving its use for only the highest-risk patients.

To better understand the role of calcium in the body, consider this:

- *Normal* deposits of calcium occur only in bone and teeth.
- *Abnormal* deposition of calcium in the body occurs in three places: the intima, the innermost layer or lining of the arteries that causes atherosclerotic plaque; the heart valves; and the medial calcification, which is the muscle layer of the arteries.

Studies also show that people with coronary disease, in conjunction with reduced blood levels of vitamin K2, show *more advanced* atherosclerotic plaque. It also appears that calcium is an active participant in the buildup of coronary plaque—and not the innocent bystander once supposed!

In a second study, Dr. Vermeer found that a diet high in both vitamins K1 and K2 could prevent and reverse Coumadin-induced arterial calcification in rats. The rat arteries that were studied resembled human arteries affected by common diabetic and age-related sclerosis (hardening of tissues).

Traditionally, calcification has been thought to be an irreversible end-stage process in arterial disease. There is a very real possibility that a vitamin supplement could roll back the sclerosis that destroys the arteries. Imagine what this could mean to individuals with diabetes and heart disease.

Could it be that many detrimental physical processes associated with age are *not* part of the so-called normal aging process? More and more, the answer is yes, and many of the pillars supporting the "carved in stone" scientific beliefs are toppling. As this information demonstrates, many of these processes can actually be reversed—and, equally important, prevented altogether.

The calcium link between arteries and bone is fascinating to me. One of the biggest tragedies of aging is osteoporosis, which predisposes us to weakness, frailty, and dangerous bone fractures, greatly limiting our mobility. Unfortunately, the calcium that belongs in our bones is transferred to arterial walls, predisposing us to cardiovascular disease and more. Adequate intake of vitamin K2 can stop this from occurring. We now have what appears to be a highly effective strategy to keep bones strong and arteries free of dangerous plaque. As you can see, **strategies that can keep bones healthy have significant impact on our cardiovascular systems as well—absolutely critical information for women with each passing decade.**

Although it is breast cancer that puts the fear of death into women, the fact is that women have a much greater chance of dying of heart disease. Vitamin K2 can greatly reduce your odds of developing this disease. Although heart disease was thought of as a "man's disease" in the past, it is the leading cause of death for both women and men in the United States, and women account for 52.6 percent of the total heart disease deaths. In 2005, heart disease was the cause of death in more than 454,000 females. Heart disease is often perceived as an "older woman's disease," and it is the leading cause of death among women age 65 and older. The fact is that heart disease is the third leading cause of death among women age 25 to 45 and the second leading cause of death among women aged 45 to 64. Remember that many cases of heart disease can be prevented!

The graph opposite shows how breast cancer compares with other common causes of death in women of all ages.

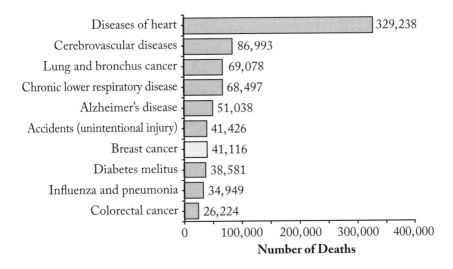

TOP TEN CAUSES OF DEATH FOR WOMEN
IN THE UNITED STATES

Source: Surveillance, Epidemiology, and End Results (SEER) Program (www.seer
.cancer.gov) SEER*Stat Database: Mortality—All COD, Public-Use with State, Total
U.S. (1969–2005), National Cancer Institute, DCCPS, Surveillance Research Program,
Cancer Statistics Branch, released February 2008. Underlying mortality data provided
by CDC's National Center for Health Statistics. For more information and facts, visit
the CDC's Heart Disease site. http://www.cdc.gov/heartdisease/.

As you can see, you are eight times as likely to die of heart disease than
breast cancer. Not to downplay the breast cancer risk, but you are also
more likely to die from an accident than you are from breast cancer!
I personally find this lack of awareness by many women about their
most dire health threat a matter of great concern.

According to the American Heart Association, nearly 37 percent of
all female deaths in America occur from cardiovascular disease. Many
women simply do not understand the dangers of heart disease and
stroke. Keeping this in mind, we take stock of the promising heart and
vascular research on Pycnogenol to date.

PYCNOGENOL SUPPLEMENTS: GOOD FOR THE BONES, GOOD FOR THE HEART

No chapter on bone health would be complete without an understanding of the nutritional supplement Pycnogenol. More than 230 scientific articles and clinical trials over the past forty years have confirmed Pycnogenol's safety, absence of toxicity, and clinical efficacy. Today, Pycnogenol is one of the most researched ingredients in the natural marketplace. Published findings have demonstrated Pycnogenol's beneficial effects in cardiovascular health, osteoarthritis, skin care, cognitive function, diabetes, inflammation, sports nutrition, asthma and allergy relief, and menstrual disorders, among others.

Pycnogenol is a natural plant extract from the bark of the maritime pine tree, which grows exclusively along the coast of southwest France in Les Landes de Gascogne.

Lowering cholesterol levels is essential in maintaining a healthy heart, since high cholesterol can increase the risk factors for atherosclerosis, heart attack, and stroke. A University of Texas, Dallas, clinical study recorded that supplementation with Pycnogenol significantly reduced the bad (LDL) cholesterol while elevating the good (HDL) cholesterol. An additional three research studies have demonstrated these same results, bringing Pycnogenol to the forefront as a viable natural choice in managing cholesterol levels.

Dr. Ronald Ross Watson at the University of Arizona concluded in his research that subjects with mild hypertension showed a significant reduction of blood pressure in response to supplementation with Pycnogenol. Additional research confirmed that 60 percent of participants who took prescribed high blood pressure medication were able to reduce their dosage by half when they supplemented with Pycnogenol.

Pycnogenol has several key health benefits that revolve around the cardiovascular system, and it has been identified in review articles as a "polypill" for heart health. To begin, Pycnogenol's basic properties provide two important capabilities for a healthy heart, including its potent antioxidant makeup and anti-inflammatory action. A number of clinical research studies show that Pycnogenol is powerful in reducing inflammation in the body, strengthening the vascular system, lowering high blood pressure and cholesterol, and fighting the effects of smoking, stress, and other environmental risk factors on the heart.

The inability of blood vessels to generate enough nitric oxide to facilitate better blood flow and blood pressure is a cardiovascular risk factor. Studies have revealed Pycnogenol restores healthy endothelial function, which helps to maintain healthy circulation by increasing the vasodilation of blood vessels, consequently improving blood flow.

Research published in *Clinical and Applied Thrombosis/Hemostasis* demonstrated that Pycnogenol protects passengers on long-distance flights from developing thrombosis. The researchers tested in-flight ankle swelling of 200 participants on airplane flights exceeding eight hours. The passengers who supplemented with Pycnogenol experienced no instances of thrombosis. Further studies recorded less leg and ankle swelling and discomfort on long-distance flights when passengers took Pycnogenol. In addition to promoting circulation, the superstrength antioxidant helps make blood platelets more slippery, which reduces the incidence of blood clots, the main cause of heart attacks.

Pycnogenol's Role in Bone Health

A study published in the journal *Redox Report* reveals Pycnogenol's anti-inflammatory potency in improving osteoarthritis symptoms and pain and in significantly lowering plasma levels of C-reactive protein (CRP). With the disease progression of osteoarthritis, the inflammation may reach a level where it is no longer limited to the affected joint and stresses the organism, increasing the inflammatory marker CRP in the blood. This study, a joint effort between Italy's Chieti-Pescara University and the University of Münster, Germany, investigated a subset of 55 patients from a previous osteoarthritis study with 156 patients who had significantly elevated CRP levels. Treatment consisted of two tablets daily of either 50 milligrams of Pycnogenol or a placebo. Blood specimens were drawn at the beginning of the initial study and again after three months of treatment. The results showed that Pycnogenol significantly lowered CRP from an average of 3.9 milligrams per liter at baseline to 1.1 milligrams per liter, an essentially healthy level. In the placebo group, a marginally lowered CRP level was detected. Other blood parameters indicative of acute inflammation likewise decreased with Pycnogenol, such as fibrinogen (lowered by 37.1 percent) and reactive oxygen species (lowered by 29.9 percent).

Inflammation is the final common denominator of many diseases, so these findings come as no surprise. They do, however, confirm that Pycnogenol is a valuable nutrient in decreasing inflammation and protecting joint health.

Dutch Treat

The Dutch countryside is dotted with beautiful brown cows grazing on lush green pasture. Many cheeses popular in the United States are imported from Holland, including Edam and Gouda. Holland is the largest exporter of cheese in the world. Its dairy industry as a whole has a turnover of around 7 billion euros—at today's exchange rate, more than $8 billion—not bad for a country about twice the size of New Jersey.

Cheese is a good natural source of K2, and Dr. Vermeer believes that cheese consumption is one reason why the Dutch have a relatively low level of cardiovascular disease. When I spent time in the Netherlands, I was surprised to be served both cheese and chocolate for breakfast! I have to confess that I enjoyed every bite.

According to Dr. Vermeer, all cheeses contain between 7.5 and 15 micrograms of vitamin K2 per ounce. Dutch researchers don't yet know why the amount of vitamin K2 varies, but they've found it to be true even within different lots of the same type of cheese produced at the same facility. "It's the same variation whether the cheese is hard or soft," says Dr. Vermeer.

Remember this key fact: milk does not contain vitamin K2; it contains just K1. The fermentation process utilized in turning milk into cheese is responsible for the vitamin K2 content in cheese, which is the result of the specific bacteria that help ferment the cheese.

Many of us shun cheese because we fear the increase of cholesterol levels from its saturated fat content. I was delighted to discover that Dr. Sinatra, a cardiologist who takes his heart health very seriously, regularly enjoys cheese and has this to say: "You may wonder, and rightfully so, if I'm concerned about the saturated fat in cheese. To tell you the truth, I'm not. Saturated fat is a source of cholesterol, and if you eat a lot of it, your cholesterol level will rise. As you well know, I'm not a big believer in cholesterol as the sole cause of heart disease, so the fat in cheese is not a big deal for me."

Dr. Sinatra recommends 150 micrograms daily of the menaquinone-7 (MK-7) form of vitamin K2. This is the most absorbable and active form of vitamin K, and it seems to also play a key role in managing calcium. He has also consulted with Dr. Leon Schurgers, another Dutch researcher who has studied vitamin K2 for more than thirty years. On the basis of animal studies, Dr. Schurgers believes that a

150-microgram dose of MK-7 is the minimum amount needed to build bone and decalcify arteries.

There are a lot of vitamin K2 products available that contain less than 150 micrograms of MK-7. Many are made predominantly with MK-4, a less active relative of MK-7. Read product labels closely to make sure that you're getting 150 micrograms daily of MK-7—and the benefits that come with it. For my vitamin K2 recommendations, see Resources.

The research clearly points to vitamin K2's critical role in cardiovascular health and calcium usage in your body. **There is no doubt that vitamin K2 is highly effective at directing calcium into your bones, where it is needed, and away from your arteries, where it does not belong.**

Say Cheese

I love all types of cheese. However, I strongly recommend that you choose only cheeses made from the raw milk of pasture-raised animals—whether dairy cows, goats, or sheep.

One of my personal favorites is Shelburne Farms three-year cheddar. On the beautiful shores of Lake Champlain in Burlington, Vermont, all the milking cows in their purebred herd of Brown Swiss are raised on the farm and graze on pasture from spring to fall. Their own milk—absolutely fresh, untreated, and rbST/rbGH free—is used to make their award-winning cheese. The only other cheese ingredients are starter culture, rennet, and salt.

Though there is some controversy regarding the safety of raw milk cheeses, if they are made from full-fat, unprocessed milk from pasture-fed cows, sheep, or goats, I believe that they are safe and superior to pasteurized cheeses in many ways. The Weston A. Price Foundation has excellent information on this topic, including a wide variety of scientific papers in support of this age-old traditional way of cheese making, at www.realmilk.com.

A great many European cheeses are also made by the traditional methods, with great pride and strict adherence to ancient and wholesome methods. According to www.gourmetfoodstore.com, only the finest French and Italian cheeses earn a special certification, which I look for when I am purchasing imported cheese.

The French Paradox

We all know that "French women don't get fat." Yet the French love their wine, and they love their cheese—two reasons that could help account for their lower rates of heart disease. I also believe that the traditional European cheeses, made from pasture-raised animals, have a much healthier profile—as do Europe's milk, meat, and butter. This is the traditional method of producing these wholesome foods. Once agribusiness started tampering with these methods, the health of people began to decline as their obesity levels rose—more about this later. Whenever you read about the most famous and sophisticated French cheeses, you will usually find them certified by the label "AOC." Right away, you know that this cheese must be important to receive such recognition—even though you may not know exactly what the AOC is. First created in the fifteenth century, this French label stands for Appellation d'Origine Côntrolée, which means Controlled Label of Origin. This guarantees that the milk is from a specific geographical area, along with the cheese's production and maturity. It also follows a traditional method of producing the cheese, as well as storing and ensuring an optimal degree of humidity in the storage room and cheese counter. Representatives from the labeling agency inspect the cheese and its production in order to ensure that it follows these guidelines.

A Taste of Italy: Molto Bene!

The Italians have their own way of guaranteeing formaggio lovers that their cheese is of the highest quality. A cheese awarded the DOP is most special. DOP stands for Denominazione di Origine Protetta, which means Protected Denomination of Origin. Similar to the AOC, the DOP guarantees that the milk for the cheese and its production are in a certain location in Italy. It is a mark of optimal quality and high standards. The methods of production must be traditional and follow fixed storage guidelines to ensure that the cheeses age correctly.

For more about cheese as well as fabulous recipes, see chapter 8, "The Forever Young Kitchen and Recipes."

Calcium

Over the years, heavy emphasis has been placed on calcium and bone health, especially for women, even though men also experience bone loss, albeit at about half the rate of women.

Unfortunately, the messages from many health care professionals and the media regarding the importance of healthy bones almost never exceed the barest of basics: the skeleton is made for holding you up and keeping you together. Almost all data regarding the importance of calcium and bone health are referenced only in this light. This is indeed an important function of the skeleton, but it is only part of the story. This focus has fostered a popular misconception about the role of bone health in overall health and longevity.

Functional bone health encompasses much more than skeletal strength alone. A healthy skeleton does more than just lower our fracture risk. It is intimately involved with our health as an *endocrine organ*. As such, it performs many important functions, including the production of red blood cells, immune cells (white blood cells), platelets, various growth factors, and cytokines, any of various protein molecules secreted by immune system cells that serve to regulate the immune system. Bone health also exerts an endocrine influence on the regulation of sugar homeostasis (the state of equilibrium or balance), fat storage, energy metabolism, and more.

Bones may be the part of our body that many of us know very little about. The fact that our bones function as an endocrine organ comes as a surprise to many of my patients. If you really wish to be Forever Young, or at least as healthy and youthful as possible, we need to place a *great deal* of emphasis on maintaining healthy bone mass during each decade of life.

Bone-Building Nutrition: Calcium Is Not a Solo Act

All of the research to date demonstrates that the best result achieved by any calcium supplement is to slow the rate of bone loss—*not* increase healthy bone density, as is the popular notion. This is a serious misconception that I am now going to remedy.

A review of the scientific literature reveals that a wide range of supplemental nutrients, in addition to calcium, can contribute to the maintenance or increasing of BMD. Nowhere is this clearer than in the recent research on the additional health benefits of calcium, vitamin D, and other bone-building nutrients. Although calcium accounts for only about 2 percent of body weight, it is essential to many life-sustaining processes that go beyond the building and preservation of bone strength. It is intimately involved in the transmission of electrical impulses that control muscles and the regulation of heartbeats. Prior to the mid-thirties, the body extracts calcium from dietary sources and stores it in bones until it is released and absorbed through the gastro-intestinal tract. As we age, this process appears to become less and less efficient. The body now needs more calcium than can be provided by the intake of commonly consumed foods and more than the bones can store. This results in a progressive decline in bone health with increased risk of fracture.

Our bodies are an amazing symphony of metabolic processes played out by an elaborate orchestra of anatomical and physiological members. Keep in mind that you are made up of food, air, water, and sunshine. This underscores the importance our diet has on maintaining healthy musicians to play this biological symphony. This also underscores the importance of the anti-inflammatory diet, the cornerstone of the entire Perricone program, which is critical to the health and optimal functioning of all organ systems, with bone health no exception. Bones require calcium, and a lot of it. Focusing only on calcium is like writing a beautiful symphony and having only one instrument play its part. It would be pathetically inadequate, as is calcium alone in the bone-building symphony.

The heavy emphasis on calcium overshadows the awareness and documented importance of the other minerals and proteins involved in bone tissue production. Without protein, minerals would be unable to form the metalloproteinase matrix necessary for bone synthesis. Without protein, bones would be brittle, fragile, and nonfunctional, and serve only as the structural scaffolding of the body. A logical conclusion is that better sources of minerals, such as protein-bound forms, naturally accompanied by a wide variety of other bone-building cofactors, might be derived from plant sources.

Plant forms of minerals could offer significant beneficial options. There is emerging evidence that plant forms of calcium and other bone health ingredients provide an alternative source of more comprehensive indigenous minerals and proteins that typically occur in a plant matrix along with other phytochemicals. Some studies have also reported positive relationships between fruit and vegetable consumption and increased BMD in adolescents as well as in adults.

A recent cross-sectional study examined the association between bone mineral status and fruit and vegetable intake in adolescent boys and girls ages 16–18, young women ages 23–27, and older men and women between the ages of 60 and 83. Using DEXA measurements of bone density, the researchers concluded that higher fruit and vegetable intakes may have positive effects on bone mineral status in adolescents and older women, especially at the spine for girls and older women and at the femoral neck for boys. Additionally, plant foods provide critical natural anti-inflammatories in the form of antioxidants. Unfortunately, the indications are that fruit and vegetable intake by the younger age groups is generally very low, and the results of the current study show that a considerable enhancement of bone mineral content (BMC) could be achieved with increased fruit and vegetable intake. *The size of the effect in the older women was impressive: doubling their fruit intake would have resulted in a 5 percent increase in spine bone mineral content.* The particular strengths of this study were the rigorous method used to assess fruit and vegetable consumption. The study analyzed the actual portion weights of fruit and vegetables, rather than the frequency of dietary intake of these two food groups or past consumption data.

On the basis of the merits indicated by the studies, which clearly demonstrate that plant forms of minerals may be more easily and efficiently used by the body, improved bone health outcomes should be expected by incorporating the three components of the surgeon general's "call to action": that is, increased nutrients, physical activity, and health literacy. Instead of utilizing combinations of isolated stand-alone inorganic rock, bone, or shell forms of minerals (calcium carbonate, calcium phosphate, and so on) or their laboratory-synthesized (chelated) versions, I recommend that we substitute pristine whole-plant forms of calcium, along with other mineral cofactors and indigenous naturally occurring phytocompounds. For example, certain species of marine algae are an abundant, naturally occurring plant form of calcium, magnesium, and a wide range of other minerals.

The ideal forms of minerals for bone health appear to be those in a pristine natural "food-type" state and therefore the most "user-friendly" for the body—in other words, compounds that are highly absorbable, usable, and beneficial. The nutrients we ingest should impose the least metabolic impact, burden, and/or consequences on the body's attempt to break them down, absorb them, and utilize them. Importantly, they would be the minerals that can produce beneficial results in improving healthy bone function. Minerals such as calcium, bound to organic ligands (citrate, malate, aspartate, lactate, alpha-ketoglutarate, etc.), have been promoted as superior to the types from rocks, shells, or bone, since we generally don't eat the latter forms. The data supporting this premise are based mostly on disintegration, dissolution, and/or poorly designed bioavailability tests and are therefore inconclusive.

From a practical standpoint, measurable beneficial effects are more important than controversies regarding absorbability and/or bioavailability. Bioavailability alone is subject to a number of variables and is therefore basically irrelevant. In the final analysis, tangible and measurable effects, such as bone density, overall health, and improved quality of life, are the most important parameters in determining the best forms of minerals. More studies are needed to investigate the therapeutic effects of plant forms of minerals over their bone, rock, shell, or synthetically reacted counterparts. I firmly believe in the superiority of plant-based forms of minerals for the reasons I have explained in this section.

Health from the Sea

What is this magic bullet we are talking about, and where can we find it? This very special gift from the sea is called *Algas calcareas*. This marine plant washes up on the pristine shores of a remote area of South America, where it is harvested by hand in waist-deep water. A team of trained locals live-harvest these marine algae from the beaches at low tide to ensure that all of the minerals and nutrients are intact. The crop is rotated from beach to beach to be sure that it does not interfere with the natural growth cycle of marine algae.

The algae are washed with fresh deionized water, sun-dried, and then milled down to powder form to become AlgaeCal. I have been extremely impressed by AlgaeCal, which has led to my working with colleagues including Dr. Harry Preuss of Georgetown University Medical School on a comprehensive peer-reviewed study to confirm its many benefits, Bone Mineral Density (BMD) Changes in a Bone Health Plan Using Two Versions of a Bone Health Supplement: A Comparative Effectiveness Research (CER) Study, currently under review for publication.

These powdered marine algae contain an entire spectrum of plant nutrients and large quantities of calcium and magnesium, plus seventy-three trace minerals. All batches of AlgaeCal powder are tested for microbial activity and mineral content to ensure quality and safety. There is no chemical treatment, no sieving process, and no additives or extractions that might create impurities. AlgaeCal is a completely natural product.

It is also the first calcium supplement to earn the certified organic classification. One of the reasons I am particularly impressed with this substance is its holistic nature; it is a whole-food calcium source as opposed to a single-element calcium source. In addition, it is from a plant source, made by nature, as opposed to an inorganic (e.g., limestone) or laboratory product. It makes much more sense to ingest a substance that is compatible with our bodies. We have been designed to accept plant minerals better than rock minerals because plants predigest the minerals for us.

Let's examine what makes AlgaeCal so special—what is in it and why it is important. As mentioned, it is a superior source of calcium, one that our body can put to work to ensure a healthy immune system and healthy bones. AlgaeCal is also an excellent source of magnesium. The Web site www.algaecal.com provides an excellent and comprehensive analysis of all of the important minerals found in this wonderful supplement and why they are so critical to our health.

Magnesium

As the fourth most abundant mineral in the body, magnesium is essential to our good health. Approximately half of our total body magnesium is found in our bones, and the other half is distributed throughout the cells of our body tissues and organs. This essential mineral is needed for more than three hundred biochemical reactions in the body. It helps maintain normal muscle and nerve function, keeps the heart rhythm steady, supports a healthy immune system, and keeps the bones strong.

Only 1 percent of magnesium is found in our blood, but the body works very hard to keep the blood levels of magnesium constant. Magnesium also helps regulate blood sugar levels, promotes normal blood pressure, and is known to be involved in energy metabolism and protein synthesis. Magnesium also plays a role in preventing and managing hypertension, cardiovascular disease, and diabetes.

Magnesium Deficiency: We Are All at Risk

According to the 1999–2000 U.S. National Health and Nutrition Examination Survey, a significant number of adults in the United States do not consume the recommended amounts of magnesium.

Research done throughout the world shows that the U.S. RDA for magnesium is not sufficient to make up for the amount lost in bowel movements and sweat. Aggravating matters more, sports, physical work, mental exertion, competition, and other stressors all increase your magnesium requirements.

To make matters even worse, the average American diet supplies even less than the RDA. Our daily magnesium intake is seriously inadequate to maintain equilibrium in metabolic balance studies. For many people, dietary intake may not be high enough to create an optimal magnesium status, which may be protective against such disorders as cardiovascular disease and immune dysfunction.

When Can Magnesium Deficiency Occur?

If your digestive system or kidney function is compromised, it can significantly influence magnesium status because magnesium is absorbed by the intestines and then transported through the blood to cells and tissues.

The bioavailability of magnesium is reasonable, with one-third to one-half of dietary magnesium being absorbed into your body. Gastrointestinal disorders that impair absorption, like Crohn's disease, can limit the body's ability to absorb magnesium. Such disorders can deplete your stores of magnesium and may result in magnesium deficiency.

Chronic or excessive vomiting and diarrhea may also result in magnesium depletion. It is interesting to note that healthy kidneys limit the urinary excretion of magnesium to compensate for low dietary intake. However, some medications cause excessive loss of magnesium in urine as a side effect. Also, poorly controlled diabetes and alcohol abuse cause the body to lose excessive amounts of magnesium.

What Is the Best Way to Get Extra Magnesium?

You can do so by eating a variety of whole grains, legumes, and vegetables (especially dark green, leafy vegetables containing chlorophyll) to increase your dietary magnesium intake. Fish such as halibut is an excellent source, as are spinach, black beans, and pumpkin and squash seeds.

Magnesium supplements may be recommended by your physician; however, taken alone, they may cause diarrhea. A more balanced approach is to take magnesium with your calcium supplement, as the two minerals work together in several ways to maintain balance. It is always best to get any mineral from a food, which is why I recommend AlgaeCal, as it naturally contains a balance of magnesium, calcium, trace minerals, and phytonutrients in a whole-food complex.

If you have low blood levels of magnesium, it is important that you have the cause, severity, and consequences evaluated by your doctor. If you have kidney disease, you may not be able to excrete excess magnesium and should not consume magnesium supplements unless they are prescribed by a physician.

Thanks to its calming effects on the nervous system, magnesium can help ease anxiety, relax muscles, promote stress relief, decrease levels of the stress hormone cortisol, and promote a good night's sleep.

Vitamin D

Vitamin D is a fat-soluble vitamin that functions as an important hormone. Vitamin D communicates to the intestines to increase the absorption of calcium by as much as 80 percent. Vitamin D is also well known for maintaining normal calcium levels. These are just a few of the extremely important functions of this essential nutrient.

Vitamin D Deficiency

In March 2006, *Mayo Clinic Proceedings* printed an alarming article about the high prevalence of vitamin D deficiency. The highly respected author, Michael Holick of the Boston University School of Medicine, stated, "Vitamin D inadequacy has been reported in approximately 36 percent of otherwise healthy young adults and up to 57 percent of general medicine inpatients in the United States and even higher percentages in Europe. Low sunlight exposure, age-related decreases in vitamin D synthesis in our skin, and diets low in vitamin D contribute to the high prevalence of vitamin D inadequacy."

Supplemental doses of vitamin D (taken together with calcium and magnesium) and sensible sun exposure could prevent deficiency in most of the general population, according to Holick. In this section we will learn which forms of vitamin D are most effective, starting with the most natural: the sun.

Vitamin D Sources

Sunlight is the best source of vitamin D. It can provide you with your entire vitamin D requirement. Children and young adults who spend a short time outside two or three times a week will generally synthesize all the vitamin D they need. If you are older, you have diminished capacity to synthesize vitamin D from sunlight exposure. Many of us use sunscreen and/or wear protective clothing in order to prevent skin cancer and sun damage, depriving ourselves of vitamin D. In these instances it is important to consider getting your vitamin D from food and supplements. Vitamin D is unique among vitamins in that it can be provided to the body through food or by exposure to the sun. Sunshine is a significant source of vitamin D because ultraviolet rays from sunlight trigger vitamin D synthesis in the skin. **I recommend spending fifteen minutes a day in the sun** *without sunscreen.* **This will increase vitamin D production, known to reduce the risk of many internal cancers as well as the risk of osteoporosis.** Although sun exposure has been greatly vilified in the past decades, exposure to the sun is our most important source of this critical vitamin.

The application of sunscreen with an SPF factor of 8 reduces the production of vitamin D by 95 percent. In latitudes around 40 degrees north or 40 degrees south (Boston is 42 degrees north), there is insufficient UVB radiation available for vitamin D synthesis from November to early March. Ten degrees farther north (Edmonton, Canada), this "vitamin D winter" extends from mid-October to mid-March. According to Dr. Holick, as little as five to ten minutes of sun exposure on arms and legs or face and arms three times weekly between 11 A.M. and 2 P.M. during the spring, summer, and fall at 42 degrees of latitude should provide a light-skinned individual with adequate vitamin D and allow for storage of any excess for use during the winter with minimal risk of skin damage.

Vitamin D Supplements

There are many health benefits of vitamin D, and, as mentioned in chapter 2 and this chapter, I recommend that we get it from sunlight. However, when this is not practical, a vitamin D supplement may be a strategy to ensure adequate levels. But what vitamin D supplement is best?

Since a large body of science shows that vitamin D works closely with calcium and magnesium, it is best to take vitamin D in combination with calcium and magnesium to maintain a proper balance. Recent literature shows that most calcium supplements have too little vitamin D to be effective. And some of them use synthetic vitamin D2. A much better form is natural vitamin D3, which stays in your system longer and with greater effect.

Effects of Vitamin D Deficiency

A deficiency of vitamin D can result in the following conditions:

RICKETS   In infants and children, severe vitamin D deficiency results in the failure of the bone to mineralize. Rapidly growing bones are most severely affected by rickets. The growth plates of bones continue to enlarge, but in the absence of adequate mineralization, the weight-bearing limbs become bowed. Although fortification of foods has led to complacency regarding vitamin D deficiency, nutritional rickets is still being reported throughout the world.

OSTEOMALACIA   Although adult bones are no longer growing, they are in a constant state of turnover. In adults with severe vitamin D deficiency, the collagen bone matrix is preserved but bone mineral is progressively lost, resulting in bone pain and osteomalacia (soft bones).

MUSCLE WEAKNESS AND PAIN   Vitamin D deficiency causes muscle weakness and pain in children and adults. In a cross-sectional study of 150 patients referred to a clinic in Minnesota for the evaluation of persistent muscle and bone pain, 93 percent had vitamin D deficiency! Muscle pain and weakness were prominent symptoms of vitamin D deficiency in a study of Arab and Danish Muslim women living in Denmark. Another trial found that supplementation of elderly women with 800 IU per day of vitamin D and 1,200 milligrams per day of calcium for three months increased muscle strength and decreased the risk of falling by almost 50 percent compared with supplementation with calcium alone. This is an extremely significant finding and a compelling case for supplementation.

Risk Factors for Vitamin D Deficiency

If you are in any of the categories below, you would be well advised to get a blood test to determine your vitamin D levels.

TOTAL COVERAGE OF THE SKIN OR OVERUSE OF SUNSCREEN Osteomalacia has been documented in women who cover all of their skin whenever they are outside for religious or cultural reasons. The application of sunscreen with an SPF factor of 8 reduces the production of vitamin D by 95 percent, creating a problem similar to that of covered skin.

DARK SKIN   People with dark skin synthesize less vitamin D on exposure to sunlight than those with light skin. The risk of vitamin D deficiency is particularly high in dark-skinned people who live far from the equator.

BREAST-FEEDING   Infants who are exclusively breast-fed are at high risk of vitamin D inadequacy, particularly if they have dark skin and/or receive little sun exposure. Human milk generally provides 25 IU of vitamin D per liter, which is not enough for an infant if it is the sole source of vitamin D. Older infants and toddlers fed exclusively milk substitutes and weaning foods that are not vitamin D–fortified are also at risk of vitamin D deficiency. The American Academy of Pediatrics recommends that all infants who are not consuming at least 500 milliliters (16 ounces) of vitamin D–fortified formula or milk be given a vitamin D supplement of 200 IU per day.

AGING The elderly have reduced capacity to synthesize vitamin D in the skin when exposed to UVB radiation and are more likely to stay indoors or use sunscreen. Institutionalized adults are at extremely high risk of vitamin D deficiency without supplementation.

INFLAMMATORY BOWEL DISEASE If you suffer from an inflammatory bowel disease like Crohn's disease, you may be at increased risk of vitamin D deficiency, especially if you have had small-bowel surgery.

FAT MALABSORPTION SYNDROMES Cystic fibrosis and cholestatic liver disease impair the absorption of dietary vitamin D.

OBESITY Being overweight increases the risk of vitamin D deficiency. Once vitamin D is synthesized in the skin or ingested, it is deposited in body fat stores, making it less bioavailable if you have large stores of body fat.

A Special Message for Menopausal Women

One of the negative effects at the onset of, during, and following menopause can be bone loss. Women in these groups are more susceptible to all of the maladies associated with weakened bones due to an increase in the rate of declining bone density and the associated loss of bone health.

Getting on the Right Tract

As mentioned, our bone marrow produces both red and white blood cells. Our red blood cells carry oxygen and nutrients to every tissue in the body. Our white blood cells are the foundation of our immune system. Seventy percent to 80 percent of our lymphatic system (immune system tissue) is located in our gastrointestinal (GI) tract. The digestive system is the first and most important step in processing the nutrients we need to exist. It is estimated that the surface area of the digestive tract is similar in size to a football field. With such a large exposure, the immune system has to work overtime to prevent pathogens from entering the blood and lymph systems. On account of this function, the GI tract is the system in the body that is most at risk from foreign matter in our food and water. It is the site of important life-protecting "recognition and response" signaling and processing, both accepting and processing the beneficial food and drink while rejecting and/or disposing of the potentially toxic.

Since our bodies are composed of food processed by the digestive system, rebuilding the digestive system itself is dependent on the efficiency of this process. It is self-perpetuating, which is why the quality of food and food supplements is so important. This is also why so much of the body's lymphatic system tissue is located in the gastrointestinal tract. A healthy digestive system is essential to healthy immune function and vice versa. And a healthy digestive system is essential to good health. If our GI tract is not functioning at its best, our immune system is also struggling. As a result, declining digestive health and function lead to declining overall health. As stated previously, all of our white blood cells are made in our bones (B cells), some of which are directed to our thymus gland, the master gland of the immune system, to become T cells.

When we contemplate these intricate interactions, it soon becomes clear that the health of our bones is instrumental to our health and longevity in general. This understanding is especially important today, because there are so many toxins and contaminants in the environment and food chain. Keeping our bones and GI tract healthy is the first step to maintaining a healthy immune system, which is vital in protecting us from the epidemics and pandemics that seem to be lurking around every corner.

Red and white blood cell production alone makes maintaining optimal bone health an important requirement for optimal overall health, especially as we age. It is no coincidence that with aging, diminishing bone health is also accompanied by reduced energy, increased fatigue, an increase in digestive problems, and an increase in maladies associated with a weakening immune system. These maladies include such disorders as rheumatoid arthritis, osteoarthritis, irritable and inflammatory bowel disorders, and a host of other chronic inflammatory and degenerative problems—another excellent reason to make sure your diet is rich in high-quality probiotics and foods that are not pro-inflammatory, since pro-inflammatory foods will compound these problems.

During medical school, one of the many basic science course requirements was embryology, the branch of biology that deals with the formation, early growth, and development of living organisms. As we studied the development of the fetus from conception to four months, we learned that all of the major organs of the body, as well as muscle, bone, and other types of tissue, are derived from three basic layers of tissue within the embryo. As you will recall, I learned that both the skin and the brain are derived from the same layer of embryonic tissue, which I call the brain-beauty connection. **Bone cells and immune stem cells have a common origin and a functional relationship, just like the skin-and-brain connection known as the osteoimmune relationship.** That functional relationship is the basis for the growing field of osteoimmunology. Consider this alarming fact: it is now known that chronic immune system overexertion leads to *bone loss* and can also promote *muscle wasting* and increased *fat storage.*

This unfortunate triumvirate does not have to be inevitable. Muscle wasting/loss of muscle mass in older people is called sarcopenia. As discussed earlier, I had long suspected that there was a strong link between inflammation and sarcopenia and used it as a model to measure and compare the loss of muscle mass seen in those who diet. I was not surprised to discover that patients who suffered from sarcopenia had higher circulating levels of inflammatory markers than those who experienced less loss of muscle mass, while other parameters had insignificant differences. Those other parameters, including levels of growth hormones and sex hormones, were fairly close to the same level in both groups. In simple terms, the subjects with the greatest loss of muscle mass were in an inflammatory state. Inflammatory markers, such as C-reactive protein and cytokines such as interleukin-6, are elevated in the people who suffer the most loss of muscle mass, or severe sarcopenia.

This loss of both bone and muscle mass, in conjunction with increased fat storage, has very special disease implications that reach far beyond the obvious aesthetics. According to Navinchandra Dadhaniya, M.D., a specialist in geriatric medicine at Illini Hospital in Pittsfield, Illinois, a healthy young person's body composition includes 30 percent muscle, 20 percent fat, and 10 percent bone. A person age 75 or over may have 15 percent muscle, 40 percent fat, and 8 percent bone.

Reduced bone density, loss of bone health, osteopenia, and osteoporosis portend much greater risks to the body than the broken hip so common in the elderly. These conditions have a systemic impact, predisposing the body to other potentially very serious disorders as well. For example, in a study presented in June 2008 at the American Society of Clinical Oncology's annual meeting, researchers from Washington University reported that maintaining bone density could be a key to decreasing the spread of breast cancer.

The Weight Loss Dilemma: Bone Health Is the Ultimate Victim

As we have seen, dieting increases our levels of inflammatory markers, accelerating the loss of precious muscle mass, but that is not the only negative consequence. There is currently an epidemic of aging people who are either overweight or obese. This is especially true for women in the process of menopause. In our efforts to combat this global problem, we run the risk of an often overlooked yet extremely harmful consequence of weight loss: the adverse effect it typically has on bone mineral density (BMD), fracture risk, and functional bone health.

At any moment millions of Americans of all ages are dieting and struggling to lose weight by means of a wide variety of programs and plans. This is particularly true of women; many start radical diets as early as their teens and continue with erratic eating habits throughout the decades. The goal of most weight loss programs is to lose as much weight as possible, as quickly as possible. In virtually all major weight loss plans, whether based on weight loss pharmaceuticals, nutriceuticals, and/or calorie-, fat-, or carbohydrate-restricted diets, little or no consideration is given to the *kind*, as opposed to the *amount*, of weight that is lost in spite of the adverse, sometimes life-threatening, effects dieting can have on both muscle mass and bone health. People are obsessed with scale weight, but it is not scale weight that is of primary importance. As we saw in chapter 3, "The Metabolic Miracle," we can and will actually weigh more if our bodies are well muscled, because muscle weighs more than fat. Weight loss, including that facilitated surgically through either gastric bypass or gastric banding procedures, has repeatedly been documented as depleting bone density and increasing fracture risk.

BMD losses are particularly pronounced in middle-aged or older Caucasian women, particularly those who are thin, petite, and over 40 with a long history of dieting. This should come as a serious and startling wake-up call to women of all ages as they struggle to keep excess weight off. In a study typifying the adverse effects of weight loss, premenopausal and early perimenopausal women who were randomly assigned to a lifestyle intervention lost 3.2 kilograms (around 7 pounds) over eighteen months and experienced rates of BMD loss at the hip that were twice those of weight-stable control subjects. In another study, in spite of a daily intake of 2,000 milligrams of calcium, bone loss occurred at some sites in overweight postmenopausal women because of weight loss. The authors report that daily calcium intake of 3,400 milligrams is more likely to minimize bone loss during weight loss in postmenopausal overweight women.

Therefore, evaluation of the overall risks and benefits of weight loss in overweight women should include monitoring its effects on BMD and the potential risks for osteopenia and osteoporosis, especially for women approaching, experiencing, and following menopause. Consideration should also be given to the type, duration, and intensity of physical activity that may retard BMD loss. Perhaps most important, diets need to be focused on decreasing inflammation as opposed to overall calories, as we will see in the next chapter. This means eating adequate high-quality protein, especially cold-water fish, lean free-range poultry, and grass-fed beef and lamb; fresh fruits and vegetables; and healthy fats such as extra-virgin olive oil.

You should do your best to limit your intake of starchy foods, eliminate all sugar, refined starches like white flour, and other processed grains. The prospect of avoiding foods that are so abundant might seem daunting, but you will feel so much better when you drop these foods from your diet that you will not even miss them.

Not Just for Women

More recently, one study tested the hypothesis that weight loss in older men is associated with increased rates of hip bone loss regardless of adiposity (fat) and intention to lose weight. Higher rates of hip bone loss were found in men experiencing weight loss, regardless of body mass index, body composition, or intention to lose weight. Even among obese men (those with a body mass index greater than 30) trying to lose weight, those with documented voluntary weight reduction experienced a greater amount of hip bone loss. Loran Salamone and colleagues examined the effect of changes in body weight on BMD in normal-weight populations. They evaluated the effect of a lifestyle intervention aimed at lowering dietary fat intake and increasing physical activity to produce modest weight loss or prevent weight gain on BMD in a population of 236 healthy, premenopausal women aged 44 to 50. Dual-energy X-ray absorptiometry analyses (DEXA) of BMD at the lumbar spine and proximal femur were made before and after eighteen months of participation in the trial. The researchers found that women in the top quartile for weight loss experienced more than three times the rate of BMD loss compared with all other women.

Alarming facts such as these inspired me to write *The Perricone Weight Loss Diet,* because with the right food and supplements, you *can* lose body fat while maintaining precious bone and muscle. As you learned in chapter 3, "The Metabolic Miracle," there is one safe, proven, and effective way to lose weight; this program will not decrease muscle or bone. In all my years of studying this topic, it has proved to be extremely effective in rapidly decreasing body fat, reducing inflammation, and improving overall health.

Almost all nutritional programs targeted at weight loss are based on various types of calorie or fat deprivation tactics, which have been shown to distress bone metabolism and health. Ironically, severe calorie restriction is also one of the only modalities shown to increase life span in animals! As contradictory as this may sound, I believe that if subclinical systemic inflammation, which is the foundation of these problems, can be reduced, body fat can safely be lost without sacrificing muscle and bone.

Studies appear to indicate that the negative relationship between reduced bone health and weight loss is affected by alterations in serum hormone levels, deficient nutritional factors, impaired energy metabolism, immune system distress, the reduction of the beneficial mechanical impact of excess weight, an increase in inflammatory markers, or some combination of these factors. Speaking of inflammation, it also appears that chronic long-term inflammation can have the effect of removing calcium from the bones, weakening and shrinking them. For women, these issues become even more pronounced with the onset and completion of menopause.

Fat Reduction Surgery and Bone Health

Though it may seem extremely radical to the average person, fat reduction surgery is very real, with more and more people who are desperate to lose weight and unable to succeed now choosing this option.

The adverse effects of weight loss on bone are being exacerbated by the tenfold increase in the number of bariatric (weight loss) surgeries performed in the United States from 13,365 in 1998 to an estimated 140,000 in 2004, a rate of increase that appears to have accelerated even more from 2004 to 2007. The American Society for Bariatric Surgery estimates that 220,000 people in the United States had bariatric surgery in 2008. Of the bariatric surgeries, Roux-en-Y gastric bypass (RYGB) is the most commonly performed surgery and appears to have substantially *greater* detrimental effects on bone health. For example, a prospective study of twenty-five women found that following RYGB, calcium absorption declined by 24 to 36 percent. Another study of 230 subjects found that within the first year following bypass surgery, BMD had decreased by an average of 7 percent.

Clearly, the results of these studies indicate that people who have had bariatric surgery should be screened with bone density testing along with repeated evaluations of their bone health–building nutritional regimens. Research also shows that postoperative bariatric patients most often have lower vitamin D levels, increased parathyroid activity, and chronically higher rates of bone mineral loss than their unoperated-upon counterparts. Therefore, aside from increasing weight-bearing exercise, it is highly recommended that bariatric surgery patients increase their vitamin D3 intake.

I want to drive home the message that you must do everything naturally possible to enhance bone health and make it your most important health priority, especially if you are nearing menopause. For all of you who have a decade or more to go before menopause, now is the time to ensure that your bones are receiving optimal nutrition to protect them now and in the future. If you are a mother with daughters, even better, as you can start them on the road to improved bone and immune health, which will provide them with a strong, healthy body.

The Adverse Effects of Disease and Medications on Bone Health

A wide range of common diseases are known to decrease bone health, including insulin-dependent diabetes, rheumatoid arthritis, inflammatory bowel disease (IBD), celiac disease, anorexia nervosa/bulimia, COPD, endometriosis, hemophilia, hemochromatosis, stroke, multiple sclerosis, Parkinson's disease, spinal cord injuries, long-term immobilization, renal disease, endocrine disorders (including suppressive doses of thyroid hormones), Addison's disease, Cushing's syndrome, sarcoidosis, organ transplants, liver disease (including hepatitis and alcoholic cirrhosis), bariatric surgery, and more. As I have just shown, a number of these disorders are either caused or contributed to by declining bone health. So it appears that there is a vicious circle working here, and one in need of a powerful cease-and-desist order.

It is very disturbing that a number of popular medications being used to treat many of these disorders also contribute to bone loss. A significant body of research has found that a wide variety of medications are associated with reduced bone health in people of all ages. The list includes glucocorticoids and related immunosuppressants, antidiabetic drugs, lithium, Depo-Provera and other contraceptives, cyclooxygenase inhibitors, proton pump inhibitors (pharmaceutical antacids), total parenteral nutrition (this means not administered via the alimentary canal), aromatase inhibitors (letrozole, exemestane, anastrozole), gonadotropin-releasing hormone agonists (Lupron, Lupron Depot, LH-RH agonists, leuprolide), immunosuppressants, anticonvulsants (phenobarbital, phenytoin), cytotoxic drugs, and selective serotonin reuptake inhibitors (SSRIs), which lead to the issue of stress and depression. The stress hormone cortisol inhibits the cells that form bone. Excess cortisol also causes many other negative effects, including the storage of abdominal fat, which you will learn about in the next chapter.

While stress and excess stress-induced depression have been shown to cause loss of bone mass, antidepressant medications have been shown to cause even further significant bone loss. This is another issue of special importance to women going through menopause, who experience a greater rate of depression and its related disorders and who are prime candidates for such medications. This could be a situation where the "cure" is worse than the disease.

In addition to good nutrition, you have to learn to manage the stress that comes with living in the modern world. That is why I have included a chapter with a full yoga workout designed to balance your body and mind.

Another recent study suggests that diabetics who are being treated with thiazolidinedione, an antidiabetic drug, provided "further evidence of a possible association between long-term use of thiazolidinediones and fractures, particularly of the hip and wrist, in patients with diabetes mellitus."

Taken together, the information presented in this chapter alone, which is only a small portion of what is available in the medical and scientific literature, continues to confirm that men and women should make bone health a top priority. Women especially need to improve the menopausal transition and minimize the consequences that have become so commonplace.

Now comes the good news—saving the best for last! As you now know, the information on bone health, as stated in this chapter, is a genuine wake-up call to the importance of bone health. Almost every system of the body benefits from improved bone health. In fact, improving bone health at any age seems to be an important factor in our ability to slow the clock of aging. It is not too far a stretch to say that healthy bones are the foundation of the fountain of youth—because you can't have one without the other. But what are the best tools to accomplish this feat? Fortunately, we have some very exciting new strategies to introduce, such as vitamin K2 and AlgaeCal.

Conclusion

New and ongoing research provides exciting insights into the importance of a well-functioning skeletal system, the broader range of nutrients than calcium needed to form healthy bones, and the probable
advantages of plant-form sources of minerals rich in calcium, magnesium, and a wide range of other naturally occurring cofactors. The
profound influence of bone health on overall health and well-being
cannot be overstated, especially for women approaching, experiencing,
and having completed menopause. Healthy bones are a foundation and
prerequisite for healthy blood, strong immunity, energy, vitality, and
optimal health.

The growing body of research into plant forms of minerals demonstrates that a number of different vitamins, minerals, and cofactors are
needed to optimize bone health, enhance the body's immune system,
and reduce the body's automatic propensity to store fat. Plant forms of
minerals also contain indigenous phytonutrients that contribute to bone
health. In looking to natural, "user-friendly" forms of minerals, we may
have found the key to stopping bone loss while dramatically improving
our overall health regardless of our chronological age.

Armed with this life-changing knowledge, you can reinvigorate,
restore, and protect yourself, while giving the term "great bone structure" a whole new meaning.

Chapter Six

THE FOREVER YOUNG APPROACH TO MENOPAUSE

Although I am often referred to as an "antiaging expert" and often use the term, my goal has never been to minimize the many positive qualities that we gain with age. Optimum health, beauty, and wisdom occur when we embrace the benefits and joys that come with *healthy* aging. These attributes include the power to learn from past mistakes, helping us to build character, compassion, tolerance, and kindness, as well as enhanced spirituality.

This philosophy defines my approach to healthy menopause and beyond. Even if you have years to go before menopause or if you have experienced this change years ago, you can significantly benefit from the Forever Young strategies delineated throughout this book. We are never too young or too advanced in years to enjoy all of the benefits of supple, youthful skin, a clear mind, abundant energy, and overall good health.

Half a Lifetime

After decades of research, designing an effective program to keep us healthy and youthful has been both a labor of love and a labor of necessity. When it comes to healthy menopause, women face unique challenges as well as opportunities. My patients all report that they are responding beautifully by following the anti-inflammatory lifestyle.

Consider this fact: most women now spend *one-third to one-half of their lives* in postmenopause. The vast majority of women have no clear understanding as to what to expect from their postmenopausal years. They lack the knowledge they need to stay vital and glowing with health and energy.

For those who have read my books and seen my public television specials, you are familiar with the idea that our appearance can be a prime motivator for starting a health program. The good news is that the benefits go far beyond a rejuvenated and more radiant beauty. Taking pride in how you look means taking proper care of yourself. When you do so, your risk of developing such diseases as heart disease, diabetes, cancer, and more is greatly reduced.

Menopause and Healthy Aging

Every day, new studies are published in the fields of health, beauty, and aging that portend a brighter future in which the negative effects of aging on mind and body are greatly mitigated.

Forever Young has not just been about introducing new strategies to reverse many of the debilitating diseases associated with so-called normal aging. As a physician with more than two decades in private practice and a dermatologist who has spent more than twenty-five years studying the aging process, I can categorically state that nothing can compare with untreated menopause as a model for *accelerated* aging, although high levels of stress and diabetes come very close. Throughout these chapters, I have introduced strategies that help all of us in general, and menopausal and postmenopausal women in particular, avoid the damaging effects of aging. What I have learned and shared in this book will mitigate many of the less positive aspects of aging and menopause—both physically and mentally.

Understanding Menopause

Simply put, menopause is the time in a woman's life when menstrual periods cease, the end of the reproductive phase of a woman's life. During menopause, a woman's hormone production drops below the level necessary to continue her periods. Menopause, a normal, natural part of aging, becomes official when you have gone twelve months without a menstrual period. Menopause occurs when your ovaries no longer produce eggs. That change is accompanied by a concomitant decrease in the hormones estrogen and progesterone.

There are three different types of menopause: natural, medically induced, and what some people refer to as "cold turkey." Natural menopause is the result of normal aging. Medical menopause is the result of chemotherapy, a hysterectomy, or another medical intervention. Cold turkey menopause results from ceasing to take hormone therapy for the treatment of breast cancer or simply ceasing to take hormone replacement therapy (HRT).

Regardless of the type of menopause, the physical transition will dramatically alter a woman's physical appearance *if left untreated*. At the same time, all organ systems can experience a decline in function. The changes experienced during what can be an emotionally and physically tumultuous period all point to the same conclusion: a rapid and obvious decline.

Perhaps the most devastating part of the clinical picture is the emotional aspect of this event. My patients describe many disturbing symptoms, ranging from simple irritability to wide emotional swings, from prolonged depression to unfounded fears and anxiety. These mental states are often accompanied by many physical changes, including increased thinning of the skin, loss of facial contours, increased lines and wrinkles, increased body fat, loss of muscle mass, decreased athletic performance, decreased bone density, and loss of sexual desire. Symptoms of menopause can include the following:

- Fatigue
- Stress
- Weight gain
- Headaches
- Loss of libido (sex drive)
- Tender breasts
- Fibrocystic breasts
- Vaginal dryness
- Uterine fibroids
- Heart palpitations
- Fluid retention (edema)
- Depression
- Irritability (mood swings)
- Anxiety
- Hot flashes, resulting in flushing and redness
- Night sweats
- Joint and/or muscle pain
- Skin wrinkling
- Loss of skin tone/firmness
- Loss of skin radiance
- Forgetfulness
- Osteopenia
- Osteoporosis, bone loss, increased risk of fractures

These psychological and physical symptoms indicate measurable physiological changes and accelerated aging. An increased risk of age-related diseases, such as heart disease, including hardening of the arteries, chest pains, and high blood pressure, is among the changes.

Take Heart

After menopause, the risk of heart disease in women becomes comparable to the incidence in men. Even I was surprised to learn that heart disease kills eight times as many women as breast cancer. In fact, as we learned in chapter 2, heart disease is the leading cause of death for woman aged 65 and over. Conversely, only about one-third of women younger than 65 with heart disease die. With proper guidance, especially nutritional and lifestyle guidance, we can significantly decrease this cardiovascular risk.

Since the number of women experiencing menopause is growing significantly, physicians and scientists need to introduce effective therapeutic strategies to ensure that women do not needlessly suffer the debilitating effects of untreated menopause. Note these national and global statistics:

North American Menopause Society, 2000

- The median age of onset of perimenopause is 47.5 years.
- In the United States, there are an estimated 41.75 million women over the age of 50.
- Most women spend one-third to one-half of their life in postmenopause.
- Smoking has been identified as a cause of early menopause.
- Natural menopause occurs at the average age of 51.4 years in Western women.
- The menopausal transition lasts an average of four years.
- In 2000, there were 45.6 million postmenopausal American women; 39.9 million of them were over the age of 51.

International Menopause Society, 2004

- Half of all women over 50 will at some time have a fracture caused by osteoporosis.
- Menopausal women are up to three times as likely as men to have Alzheimer's disease, and research suggests that menopause may play a significant role.
- Recent surveys have found that more than half of all women don't know that menopause is associated with an increased risk of heart disease.

By the year 2025, the World Health Organization estimates, 1.1 billion women will be age 50 or over.

Decelerating the Aging Process

Despite the seriousness of the risks that accompany menopause, we know that we can overcome many of the avoidable illnesses resulting from the accelerated aging associated with untreated menopause. As we have learned in earlier chapters, we can help maintain radiant, healthy, and firm skin; an athletic and toned body; elevated mood; clear, logical thinking; and freedom from memory loss, maintaining the same problem-solving abilities we had in our twenties and a renewed enthusiasm for all aspects of life. *Forever Young* offers a simple and realistic approach to facing a new and different reality, one that shows you how to experience the joys of continued health, vibrancy, and beauty throughout life.

Menopause is a wake-up call to our own mortality. You will see and feel the negative effects if you don't rise to the challenge; the choice is yours. This goes too for men, who also go through a prolonged and not-so-obvious change, a male menopause known as andropause.

Making the Most of a Major Milestone

Menopause does not have to be a model for accelerated aging. Instead, it can symbolize a milestone in your life, one that motivates you to achieve a new level of health, beauty, wisdom, and spirituality. This is not hyperbole but well-researched, science-based information that can change the way you look and feel as you approach this momentous event on the biological timeline.

Menopause does not mean farewell to femininity and glamour, health and well-being. The Perricone philosophy is firmly rooted in mental and physical health and function. I often tell my patients that radiant health is true beauty. This starts with the foods we eat. In fact, I have discovered that the greatest gift I can give my readers is permission to eat healthful, delicious food. There is no more powerful medium for good or ill than our daily food choices. This simple concept is hugely empowering, because it means that the most effective health and beauty strategies are accessible to everyone, every day.

Reducing Menopausal Symptoms with Diet

I place nutrition, the foods we eat, and the beverages we drink at the very center of the *Forever Young* program. Regardless of your age, you can and will benefit from following the anti-inflammatory diet. In this book a number of outstanding foods that slow aging and also rejuvenate the body at a cellular level have been introduced. Many of my patients are surprised to learn how much power our food choices wield, and this is particularly evident when it comes to some of the common discomforts that women experience during menopause.

During this time frame a number of health concerns surface, affecting women during this stage of life and into their later years. There is a wide variation of symptoms both among women of the same culture and among women of different cultures. A common link in these differences appears to be lifestyle and diet, although as with most health concerns, genetic factors play a role as well, but a genetic predisposition to a health condition can be influenced greatly by both diet and lifestyle.

Cultural differences underscore the importance of vegetable consumption in preventing menopausal symptoms. A much lower percentage of Asian women than U.S. women experience menopausal symptoms. For example, for women over 50 years of age, hot flashes are experienced by approximately 75 percent of American women and less than 25 percent of Asian women. This dramatic difference in the occurrence of hot flashes may be attributed to differences in diet. Americans consume a diet much higher in meat and animal fats and lower in vegetables, fruits, and fiber than do Asian women. Due to dietary differences and perhaps higher activity levels as well, Asian women have a lower percentage of body fat than do American women. This contributes to a lower circulating level of estrogen, since fat cells, as well as the ovaries, produce estrogen.

Therefore, a diet high in meat and animal fat that does not come from organic, 100 percent pasture-raised animals and low in vegetables and fiber promotes higher circulating levels of estrogen in premenopausal women. This may result in more noticeable symptoms once the body ceases to produce estrogen. This contrasts with the situation of Asian women, who, because of their low intake of animal fat and high vegetable and fiber intake, have lower premenopausal circulating levels of estrogen. This means that they do not undergo as dramatic a decrease in circulating estrogen levels during menopause. Reducing the intake of animal fats and increasing that of fiber-rich vegetables (which can also help lower body fat), as well as cold-water fish, can help decrease menopausal symptoms by reducing the circulating levels of estrogen prior to the onset of menopause.

That is not all. A diet rich in plant foods provides many other health benefits, including support for digestion and liver function, cardiovascular health, bone strength, energy levels, immunity, vision, and mental function, among others. As you know, the antioxidants in plant foods act as natural anti-inflammatories. In that capacity, they are able to ameliorate a great many unpleasant symptoms associated with menopause as well as aging in general.

See page 259 for specific dietary guidelines.

Fortunately, diet and lifestyle can be adjusted to help reduce, prevent, and even reverse some of the menopausal and postmenopausal symptoms. Though genetics plays a major role in determining the age of onset of menopause, diet and lifestyle are key players in determining the intensity, frequency, and duration of menopausal symptoms. Adopting dietary and lifestyle strategies to help cope with menopausal symptoms will improve overall health, vitality, and longevity. Leading nutrition and medical experts advocate daily consumption of fresh vegetables and fruits as a prerequisite for good health. Fresh vegetables and fruits also contain phytonutrients and phytochemicals that I believe can help reduce menopausal symptoms as well.

Phytoestrogens

While an anti-inflammatory diet high in vegetables and healthy fats from cold-water fish, olive oil, nuts, and seeds (especially chia seeds) and low in animal fat can help lower body fat and premenopausal estrogen levels, vegetables are also a source of certain phytochemicals known as phytoestrogens that may help lessen menopausal symptoms. Phytoestrogens, chemicals found in hundreds of different plants, have a structural similarity to estrogen. Understanding the role of phytoestrogens in women's health is of particular importance in this chapter because it is a key factor in health and well-being both during menopause and beyond. Understanding the different sources of phytoestrogens and how they work in the body is critical in making the right choices. Supermarkets, drugstores, and natural food market shelves are filled with myriad products from supplements to foods, protein bars, and drinks directed at women with claims about their targeted health benefits. Unfortunately, many women make choices based on the extensive marketing and advertising that these companies pay for rather than on a clear understanding of the products' mechanism of action.

Mechanism of Action

Phytoestrogens bind to estrogen receptors and may exhibit weak estrogenic or antiestrogenic effects. Phytoestrogens do not have the same ability that estrogen has when it comes to effecting changes mediated by the estrogen receptor. The small effect that phytoestrogens do have appears to help offset some of the more common menopausal symptoms. These include hot flashes, irritability, mood swings, and sleep disturbances. Studies also suggest that phytoestrogens may play a role in preventing the occurrence of chronic diseases during postmenopause, including coronary heart disease, atherosclerosis, hypercholesterolemia, cancer, and osteoporosis.

Soy and Flaxseed: The Pros and Cons

Both laboratory and clinical studies indicate that phytoestrogens provide health benefits during both menopause and postmenopause. These include protecting cardiovascular health by lowering levels of blood cholesterol and increasing the strength and elasticity of blood vessels, inhibiting the onset and progression of cancer, and conserving bone mass. In this regard, two major sources of phytoestrogens have been the focus of epidemiological studies: soy and flaxseeds. Soy and flaxseeds have both been reported to reduce the frequency and intensity of hot flashes during menopause. They have also been reported to decrease rates of cardiovascular disease, cancer, and osteoporosis during postmenopause.

Isoflavone phytoestrogens such as genistein from soy and certain lignan phytoestrogens may protect against the possible carcinogenic actions of estrogen by:

- Inhibiting the production of estrogen by the enzyme aromatase, which is responsible for a key step in the biosynthesis of estrogens
- Competing at the estrogen receptor level, with either estrogen or xenoestrogens (industrial and agricultural chemicals such as bisphenol-A and pesticides), which have potent estrogen-like and carcinogenic activities

Preventing overstimulation of estrogen receptors and providing low-level estrogen stimulation help prevent the negative effects of estrogen while providing a beneficial lower level of estrogen stimulation.

There is somewhat of a catch-22 to this scenario. Some isoflavones from soy may actually *increase* estrogen activity rather than inhibit it. These opposing effects of different soy phytoestrogens may be responsible for reports of both negative and beneficial actions of soy on women's health. Using soy is somewhat controversial, and it may be safer to avoid soy and soy-based products.

Estrogen is produced in a series of enzymatically controlled biochemical reactions. Aromatase is a key enzyme that converts testosterone into estrogen. The good news is that, at low concentrations, phytoestrogens have been found to inhibit aromatase activity, lowering estrogen production and estrogen-related changes in the body. At high concentrations, phytoestrogens may mimic the effects of estrogen. Inhibition of aromatase at low concentrations may contribute to the reported anticancer effects of phytoestrogens.

The plant lignans secoisolariciresinol diglucoside (SDG), matairesinol, and pinoresinol in flaxseeds are converted in the colon of humans and other animals into the mammalian lignans enterodiol and enterolactone, which are more potent phytoestrogens than plant lignans. Enterodiol and enterolactone are called mammalian lignans because bacteria synthesize these lignans in the mammalian colon from plant lignans. They are found only in mammals, not in plants.

This is another important reason why we need to keep the natural flora in our colon intact by eating the right foods and supplements that supply both probiotic bacteria, such as that found in plain unsweetened yogurt and kefir, and the fructooligosaccharides that the bacteria feed on.

Chia Seeds Versus Flaxseeds

Though almost all research on lignans has centered on flaxseed lignans, there are concerns regarding the content of cyanogenic glycosides in flaxseeds and the potential for oxidation of ground flaxseed powder and flaxseed oil. Chia seed, which contains the *same or higher* levels of lignans as flaxseed, has no known toxins, is resistant to oxidation (a key point), and may be preferable to soy and flaxseeds as a safe, effective source of phytoestrogens.

Chia Seeds, a Remarkable Superfood

I introduced chia seeds in chapter 3, "The Metabolic Miracle," and re-introduce them here as an important food to eat during menopause. As with any food, especially food eaten specifically for health reasons, it is best to consume those with organic certification. One of the few organic chia seed products on the market is Green Foods organic chia seeds. This is made from organic chia seeds grown in fertile, organic soil in an ideal subtropical climate that provides the best possible conditions for growth and nutrient content, eliminating the need for herbicides, fungicides, or pesticides. Organic chia seeds from Green Foods Corporation also contain many other nutrients, including vitamin E; minerals for bone support; high-quality protein; a perfect balance of omega-3, -6, and -9 fatty acids; and soluble fiber for gentle internal cleansing and digestive support.

Omega-3s and Hot Flashes

For many years, hormone replacement therapy (HRT) has been the only reliably effective treatment for hot flashes, but unfortunately it may pose real risks. The good news is that the results of a new trial, reported in the Vital Choice newsletter and generously shared here, supports prior indications that omega-3 fish oils may substantially reduce hot flashes.

> While several nonprescription treatments—isoflavones and black cohosh, for example—have shown promise in preliminary investigations, none possess conclusive evidence of efficacy. One challenge facing any alternative to HRT is that hot flashes respond to placebo (inactive) treatments more strongly than most medical conditions do.
>
> Accordingly, any proposed treatment for hot flashes has to be highly effective to improve on the very strong placebo effect seen in most clinical trials. . . .
>
> CANADIAN TRIAL FINDS OMEGA-3s
> MAY FIGHT HOT FLASHES
>
> Dr. Michel Lucas and his colleagues at Quebec's Université Laval recruited 120 women aged 40 to 55 and divided them into two groups.
>
> When the study started, the average number of daily hot flashes experienced by all of the women was 2.8.
>
> Women in the first group took fish oil capsules standardized to provide one gram of EPA—one of the two key omega-3s in fish oil—every day for eight weeks.
>
> Women in a second, "control" group took capsules containing sunflower oil free of EPA. The women taking omega-3 EPA reported 1.58 fewer daily flashes, compared with only 0.5 fewer flashes in the control group, taking sunflower oil.

The researchers found that the odds of experiencing positive results were about three times greater among those taking EPA than among those taking the placebo. The Canadians did qualify their results, saying their findings needed to be confirmed by a clinical trial specifically designed to evaluate hot flashes in more symptomatic women. **What is remarkable about their findings is that the decrease of 1.1 hot flashes per day that they attributed to the use of omega-3s is equivalent to results obtained with hormone therapy and antidepressants.**

To conclude, I want to assure you that menopause is not synonymous with loss. Menopause does not have to herald a precipitous decline into old age. It is a time of transition, like adolescence, except now you have the experience and power to move through these changes with grace and serenity. *Forever Young* has given you the tools to manage your menopause, to reduce, prevent, and reverse some of your symptoms so that you can live life to the fullest.

In the following chapter we will explore the physical and mental revitalization that practicing yoga can produce—just a few simple yoga poses a day will result in wonderful and very visible benefits regardless of your age or physical condition.

Chapter
Seven

YOGA FOR BEAUTY, HEALTH, AND LONGEVITY

To my mind, the benefits of yoga are unparalleled. Back in 2003, when I was writing *The Acne Prescription*, later renamed *The Clear Skin Prescription*, I was faced with a dilemma because certain types of exercise can cause acne to worsen dramatically. For example, lifting heavy weights and weight training can actually make acne worse. Regardless of gender, these forms of exercise make us much more susceptible to acne breakouts. The reason is simple: weight lifting and weight training increase levels of our male hormones, such as testosterone, which can contribute to acne.

Exercising too strenuously or for too long can also be detrimental. Obviously, we can't let our muscles atrophy, which they will do if we don't perform some sort of weight or strength training. The key is *moderate* exercise, a vital component of any healthy lifestyle.

Typical Western forms of exercise are designed to make your heart and lungs work hard. The principal aims of this kind of exercise are building good muscle tone, burning fat, and increasing endurance. Though these goals are worthy and important, we need to be careful when performing vigorous physical exercise. Too much exertion increases oxygen demand beyond the optimum level. This causes the production of inflammatory free radicals, and you know what that means. Ironically, the wrong type of exercise will backfire by accelerating the aging process. Though there is a vital role for aerobic types of exercise, it is important that they not be overdone.

The right exercise will strengthen your bones and muscles, improve and restore your physical and emotional balance, promote cellular rejuvenation on all levels, increase strength and flexibility, relieve stress, and improve physical, mental, and emotional health. To achieve these goals, we need to incorporate specific types of exercise. Disciplines such as yoga, tai chi, and chi kung may not seem strenuous enough, yet they yield unparalleled physical, mental, emotional, and spiritual benefits. That is why I dedicated chapter 7 to a yoga workout.

If you are wondering how this might be relevant to you, let me explain. In conjunction with poor nutrition, stress is the single greatest precipitator of premature aging, and exercise is the most effective way to reduce stress. In order to stay Forever Young, meditation or some form of effective relaxation is necessary to lower stress levels. Yoga, which combines exercise with meditation, has been shown to reduce stress levels.

Yoga provides a superior form of meditation, but yoga is not a passive meditation. A twenty-minute yoga session will leave you relaxed yet physically invigorated, with a strong sense of well-being. It is the perfect antidote for people who lead busy, stress-filled lives, and want to look and feel their best. I have also observed that a great many yoga practitioners look significantly younger than their chronological age, in both face and body.

To showcase the many benefits of yoga in *The Clear Skin Prescription*, I went to the experts. Trisha Lamb Feuerstein of the International Association of Yoga Teachers generously gave me permission to reprint

the impressive list of "Health Benefits of Yoga" that appears at www
.iayt.org. I recommend that you visit this excellent site.

Forever Young is the perfect venue in which to reintroduce yoga,
because the benefits of yoga are unparalleled at every age. My goal has
always been to present holistic solutions that work. Yoga is unique in
that it addresses the entire person:

- It exercises and tones the body.
- It energizes yet soothes the mind.
- It helps the practitioner achieve a deeply meditative state.

In *Forever Young,* I am also fortunate to showcase another expert,
Wini Linguvic, who has a long history as an incomparable yoga in-
structor and celebrity trainer. Wini also enjoys a deep understanding
of yoga's capacity as a healing art. Consistent practice strengthens the
body, mind, and spirit—the ideal antidote to the stresses of today's
world.

Radiant Strength for Radiant Health

As true beauty is the manifestation of radiant health, it is also the manifestation of physical strength. The routines Wini creates for her clients
combine multiple aspects of fitness, drawing from strength training, core
conditioning, and both traditional and modern yoga methods. The program she has designed for *Forever Young* increases strength, flexibility, and
overall conditioning in a series of specifically designed yoga sequences.

As Wini says, we are all already strong. The poses and exercises we
practice simply uncover the strength that is already there, waiting to be
uncovered. This should come as good news to all of you who have never
tried yoga, thinking that gymnastic skill is necessary. In fact, nothing
could be farther from the truth. When in the hands of an expert such
as Wini, yoga becomes not only accessible but empowering.

Workouts that integrate yoga with conditioning moves provide a multitude of benefits, including a decreased risk of injury, improved posture, the ability to carry your own weight, and a significant increase in the overall quality of life. Yet it is the unseen rewards that repay the investment of just a few hours a week.

As a teacher, Wini wants to ensure that we learn that we can get stronger, that a movement that was once seemingly impossible is approachable, and that a pose that was once difficult is now a powerful tool for reducing stress, all of which give us a sense of control over our lives. We learn, through consistent training, that we can control the way we feel, that we can improve on a new skill, that we can calm our mind and body. *The knowledge that we have control over our inner landscape is priceless.*

Outlined here is Wini's program for *Forever Young* readers, ideal at any age and particularly helpful for women near menopause, during menopause, and postmenopause.

WINISM BY WINI LINGUVIC

A note on tailoring your program: choose what is appropriate for you. There are thousands of yoga poses for a reason; although not everyone should do every pose, there are poses for everyone. The key is to forever be the student, balancing between listening to your body and searching for challenges to take you to the next level.

Yoga to Recharge and Regenerate

The word *yoga* comes from Sanskrit and means "to yoke" or "to unite." This can mean uniting mind and body. Yet the word *unite* can go beyond that to encompass the merging of soft and strong, breath and movement, grace and strength.

Benefits

Uniting of Mind and Body

Yoga offers the opportunity to delve deeper into the body. When you remain in a yoga pose, you focus on your breath and how your body is responding. The beauty of yoga is that you can always go deeper: the poses often remain the same; what changes is you.

Most of our lives, whether we are working, reading, or just taking care of our families, we need to have an alert mind. Our bodies are often a mere afterthought; we adjust ourselves in our chairs or cars and focus on our minds. Yoga offers the opportunity to wake up the body, to bring a sense of alertness and awareness to our physical self.

Softness and Strength

Yoga also requires you to be both soft and strong. The *Yoga Sutra,* an ancient text on yoga, refers to *sthira sukham asanam,* which suggests that each pose should be both steady and comfortable. A pose as simple as Downward-Facing Dog requires you to be fully present in your body yet soft in breath and mind. There are layers of awareness in each pose, and with each practice you have the opportunity to balance the opposites of soft and strong. This learning to deal with opposing forces can reach beyond your yoga practice into all aspects of your life.

Breath and Movement

Yoga links breath to the movements of the body, requiring you to focus on the moment. As each movement matches your breath, your mind quiets, allowing you to delve deeper into yourself.

A Sense of Control

The true value of yoga is recognizing that yoga is a tool for healing. In an ever-changing world, where so many things are out of our control, knowing that you have access to a toolbox of poses and exercises to improve your well-being provides a sense of control. When you know that you have an arsenal of tools, simple yoga poses and sequences that quiet your mind and revive your body, the everyday challenges are not so overwhelming.

Regular yoga practice allows us to tune in to what is going on in our bodies. Dialing into our energy is a skill that comes with regular practice. It is as if we are tuning in to a radio station; we can start to listen, really listen, to what is going on inside. And knowing that we can start to sense how we are feeling, how our bodies are responding to specific yoga routines, is extremely empowering.

Bone Strength

Thirty minutes of weight-bearing exercise helps counter the effects of bone loss. Overall stress reduction can also counter some of the effects of bone loss. A yoga sequence that focuses on standing poses can be a bone builder as well as a stress buster. Weight-bearing yoga poses can increase joint mobility, lubricate the joints, and increase overall strength.

Stress Reduction

Often menopause is a time of stress; the body gets caught in a constant cycle of stress overload. Hormones rise and fall, taxing the system, and the body experiences more stress trying to catch up with itself. Incorporating a daily yoga practice with sequences to reduce stress brings your body into balance and gets you off of the stress roller coaster.

Finding the Time

A common challenge I hear from clients is that although they know they will feel better after practicing yoga, they cannot find even 15 minutes to practice. I understand how busy life gets, but the days you can't find 15 minutes are the days you need to practice for at least 30 minutes. If you start to think of yoga as adding to your day, instead of something that takes away from your time, you will always find some time during your day to recharge and regenerate.

Yoga Sequences

There are specific yoga sequences to alleviate menopausal symptoms: hot flashes, fatigue, insomnia, headaches, and depression. There are also specific yoga sequences to improve strength and conditioning.

Strengthening Sequence

This is a general overall strengthening sequence designed to increase bone density, overall strength, and flexibility and reduce stress and fatigue.

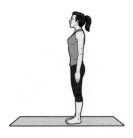

MOUNTAIN POSE (PAGE 220)

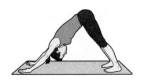

DOWNWARD-FACING DOG
(PAGE 221)

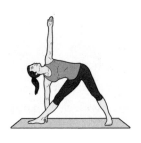

TRIANGLE POSE (PAGE 222)

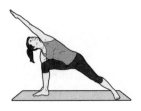

EXTENDED SIDE-ANGLE POSE
(PAGE 223)

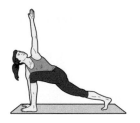

CRESCENT TWIST (PAGE 224)

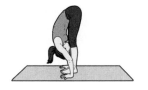

STANDING FORWARD BEND
(PAGE 225)

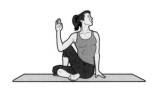

SEATED TWIST (PAGE 226)

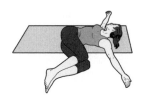

RECLINING TWIST (PAGE 227)

Core Strength Sequence

A specific sequence designed to increase core strength, which translates to better posture and stronger lower back and abdominals.

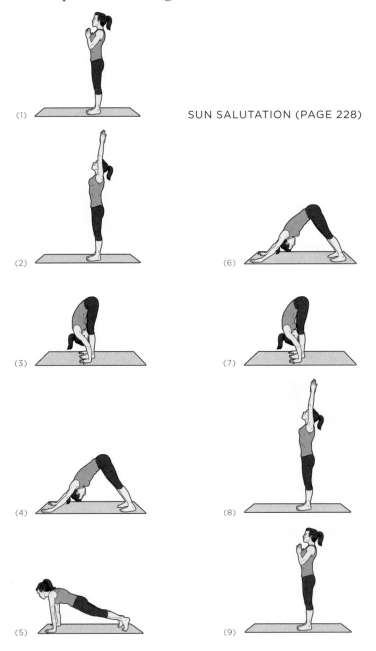

SUN SALUTATION (PAGE 228)

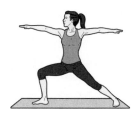

WARRIOR TWO (PAGE 231)

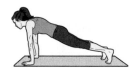

PLANK POSE (PAGE 232)

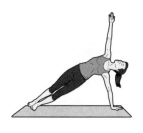

SIDE PLANK POSE (PAGE 233)

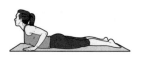

COBRA POSE (PAGE 234)

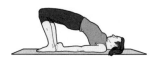

BRIDGE POSE (PAGE 241)

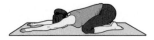

CHILD'S POSE (PAGE 250)

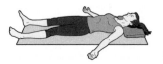

CORPSE POSE (PAGE 252)

Balancing Sequence for Hot Flashes

This sequence for reducing hot flashes includes poses that are cooling and restorative. In addition, a basic strengthening sequence will help reduce the stress and fatigue that can intensify hot flashes.

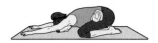

CHILD'S POSE WITH TRACTION
(PAGE 251)

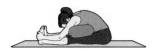

SUPPORTED FORWARD BEND
(PAGE 235)

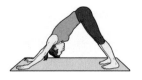

DOWNWARD-FACING DOG
(PAGE 221)

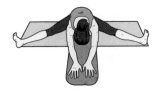

SEATED UPRIGHT WIDE-ANGLE POSE
(PAGE 236)

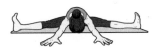

SEATED FORWARD WIDE-ANGLE
POSE (PAGE 237)

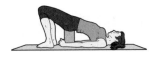

SUPPORTED BRIDGE POSE (PAGE 242)

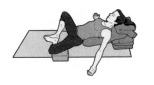

SUPPORTED GODDESS POSE
(PAGE 243)

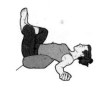

LEGS UP THE WALL POSE (PAGE 244)

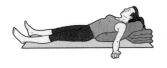

SUPPORTED CORPSE POSE
(PAGE 246)

Restorative Sequence for Stress and Fatigue

Stress and fatigue tend to intensify menopausal symptoms; yoga in general decreases stress and fatigue. This sequence can be done to relax at the end of the day.

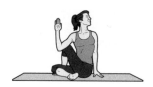

SEATED POSE (PAGE 247)

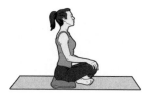

GENTLE TWIST (PAGE 248)

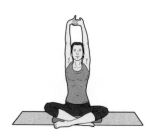

SEATED OVERHEAD EXTENSION
(PAGE 249)

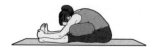

SUPPORTED FORWARD BEND
(PAGE 235)

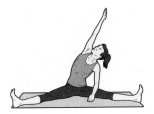

SEATED REVOLVED WIDE-ANGLE POSE

(PAGE 239)

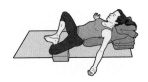

SEATED LATERAL WIDE-ANGLE POSE

(PAGE 238)

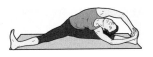

SUPPORTED GODDESS POSE

(PAGE 243)

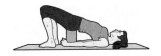

SUPPORTED BRIDGE POSE

(PAGE 242)

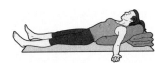

SUPPORTED CORPSE POSE

(PAGE 246)

How to Perform the Poses

MOUNTAIN POSE
TADASANA

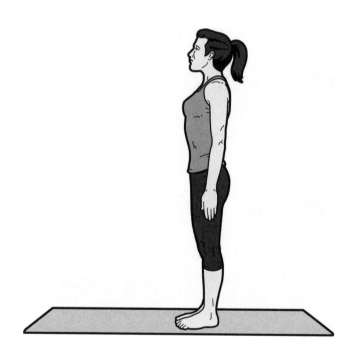

Stand with your feet parallel and hip width apart.

Place all four corners of your feet on the floor.

Lift your thigh muscles by drawing your knees up toward your hips.

Shift your weight back slightly.

Go deeper: root your feet into the floor to get a rebound effect.

DOWNWARD-FACING DOG
ADHO MUKHA SVANASANA

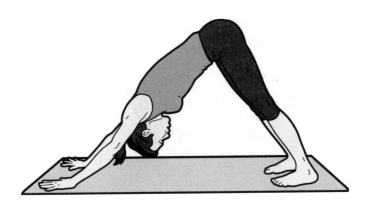

Go onto the floor on your hands and knees.

Place your knees directly below your hips and your hands slightly in front of your shoulders.

Press your palms onto the floor and tuck your toes under.

Exhaling, lift your knees away from the floor and extend your legs.

Press the knuckles of your index fingers down as you extend your arms.

Draw the inner edges of your shoulder blades in toward your back as you lengthen your torso toward the hips.

Press your thighs back as you draw your knees up and lower your heels toward the floor.

Breathe into the pose for five to ten breaths, working your way up to 1 to 3 minutes.

TRIANGLE POSE
TRIKONASANA

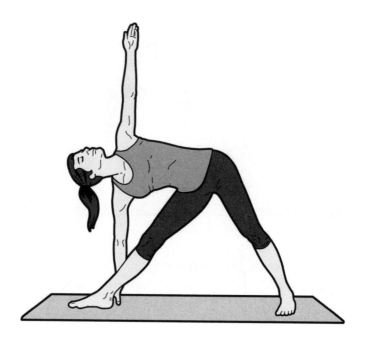

Position your feet about 4 feet apart.

Extend your arms out through your fingertips.

Turn your right foot out 90 degrees and your left foot slightly in.

On the exhale, extend your torso to the right and place your right hand on your right shin or on the floor behind your ankle.

Turn your chest to the ceiling and look to the sky.

Roll your left shoulder back and extend your left arm toward the ceiling.

Breathe into the pose for five breaths, then press your feet firmly into the floor to come up.

Switch sides and repeat.

EXTENDED SIDE-ANGLE POSE
PARSVAKONASANA

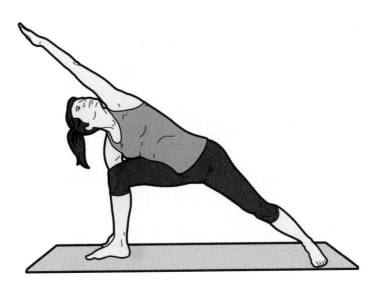

Stand in Mountain Pose (page 220).

Position your feet about 4 feet apart.

Turn your right foot and leg out 90 degrees and your left foot in slightly.

Align your right heel with the arch of your left foot.

Anchor your left heel down and draw your left inner thigh in toward your pelvis.

Bend your right leg until it is parallel to the floor with your knee in line with the ankle.

Firm your shoulder blades and extend your torso to the right, reaching your right fingertips to the outside of your right foot and extending your left arm over your ear.

CRESCENT TWIST

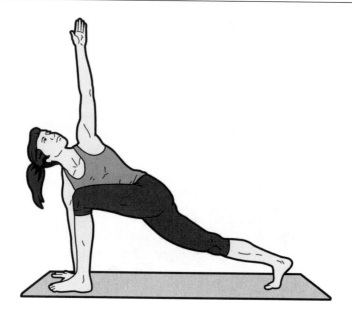

Stand in Mountain Pose (page 220).

Position your feet 4 feet apart with hands on hips.

Turn your right foot out 90 degrees and turn your left foot in so the heel lifts off the floor.

Bend your right knee until your thigh is parallel to the floor.

Rotate your torso to the right until you are facing directly over the right leg and lift your left heel as you bend your right leg so it is parallel to the floor.

Keep your left leg alert by drawing your thighbone up, hugging your tailbone in, and extending through your left heel.

Turn farther to the right and place your left hand on the floor inside your right foot. Draw your right hip back as you extend through the arms and rotate your torso to the right.

Remain for five breaths.

Switch sides and repeat.

STANDING FORWARD BEND
UTANASANA

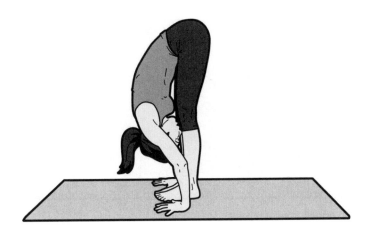

Stand in Mountain Pose (page 220).

Place your hands on your hips and firm your legs.

Exhale and bend forward with a long spine.

Place your fingertips on the floor beside your feet.

Draw your knees up, firming your thighs, and allow your torso to release down.

To come up, extend your spine into a concave position, raise your head, place your hands on your hips, and rise up with a long spine.

SEATED TWIST

ARDHA MATSYENDRASANA

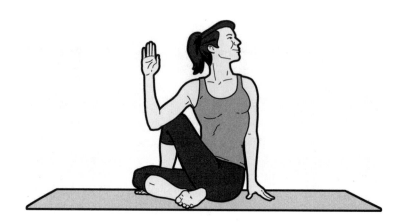

Sit on the floor with your legs extended.

Bend your knees and place your left foot under your right leg and your right foot over your left leg with your right foot pressing on the floor and your right knee pointing toward the ceiling.

Lengthen your spine and twist as you press your right hand onto the mat just behind your sacrum, and place your left arm on the outside of your right thigh.

Gently twist toward the right.

Continue to lengthen your spine with each breath.

Remain for five breaths and switch sides.

RECLINING TWIST
SUPTA MATSYENDRASANA

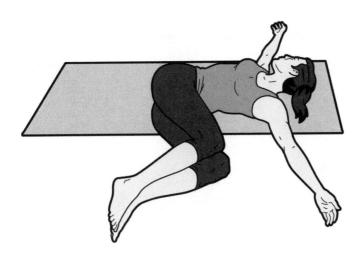

Lie on your back and hug your knees to your chest.

Move your legs to your right side.

Release your upper back and let both shoulder blades move toward the floor.

If your arm does not reach the floor, place a folded blanket underneath it.

With each exhale, sink deeper into the pose.

Stay for ten breaths, then bring the knees back to the middle.

Repeat on the other side.

SUN SALUTATION

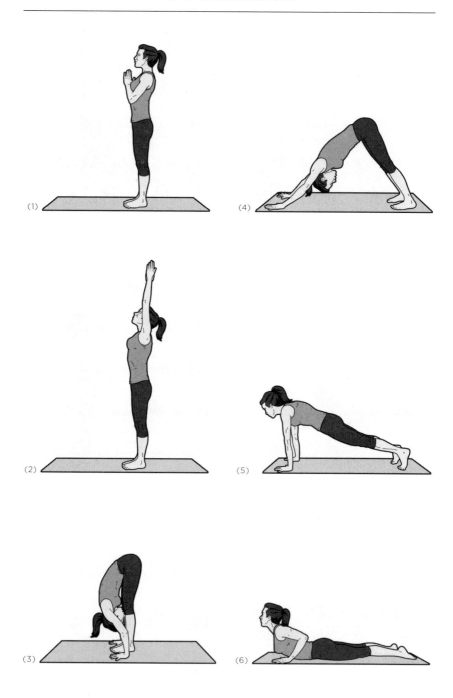

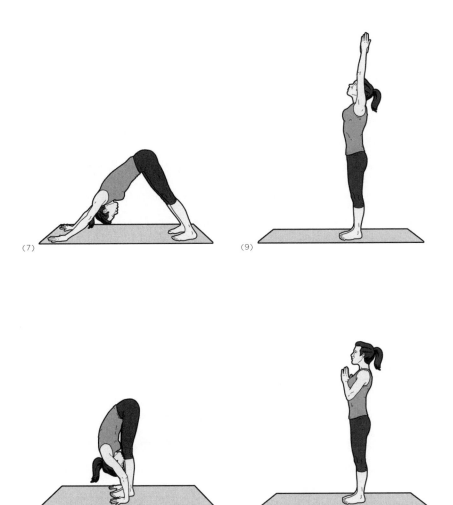

(7)   (8)   (9)   (10)

The Sun Salutation is a series of yoga poses that flow together in a moving meditation.

Stand tall with your hands in prayer.
Inhale and lift your arms overhead.
Exhale into Standing Forward Bend.
Inhale and lift the chest.

Exhale into Standing Forward Bend.

Inhale and step back into Plank Pose.

Exhale and lower yourself toward the floor.

Inhale and lift the chest into Cobra Pose.

Exhale and lift back into the Downward-Facing Dog.

Inhale and walk your feet between your hands.

Exhale into Standing Forward Bend.

Inhale and stand up, lifting your arms above your head.

Exhale and place your hands in prayer at your chest.

Repeat one to five times.

WARRIOR TWO
VIRABHADRASANA II

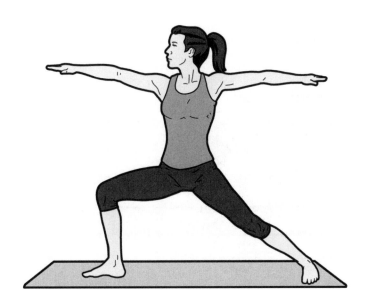

Stand in Mountain Pose.

Position your feet about 4 feet apart.

Turn your right foot and leg out 90 degrees, and turn your left foot in slightly.

Align your right heel with the arch of your left foot.

Anchor your left heel down and draw your left inner thigh in toward your pelvis.

Bend your right leg until it is parallel to the floor with your knee in line with your ankle.

Keep your torso upright as you extend your arms out.

Hug your tailbone in a bit toward your pubis.

Turn your head to the right and focus beyond your right hand.

Remain for five to ten breaths, then switch sides.

PLANK POSE

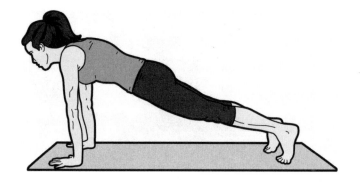

Start in Downward-Facing Dog (page 221). Then draw your torso forward until the arms are perpendicular to the floor. Your shoulders should be directly over the wrists and your abdominals should be drawn in.

Press your front thighs up as you lengthen your tailbone toward your heels.

With each exhale feel your ribs soften and your abdominals draw upward.

SIDE PLANK POSE

VASISTHASANA

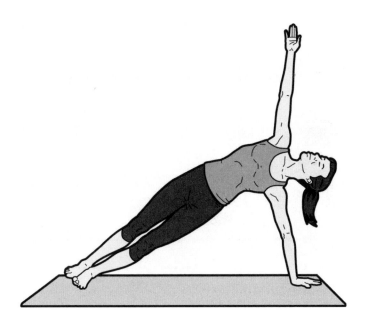

Start in Downward-Facing Dog (page 221).

Shift onto the outside edge of your right foot, and stack your left foot on top of the right.

Place your left hand onto your left hip as you turn your torso to the left.

Make sure your supporting arm is slightly in front of your shoulder.

Drawing your abdominals in, create a diagonal line from the top of your head through your heels.

Remain in the pose for five breaths.

Switch sides.

COBRA POSE

BHUJANGASANA

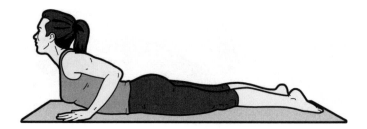

Lie prone on your mat.

Extend your legs back.

Place your hands on the floor beneath your shoulders and draw the elbows toward your sides.

Press your thighs, your hips, and the tops of your feet firmly into the mat.

Extend your arms to raise your chest off the floor.

Draw your tailbone toward your pubis as you gently lengthen your spine.

Remain in the pose for five to ten breaths.

SUPPORTED FORWARD BEND
PASCHIMOTTANASANA

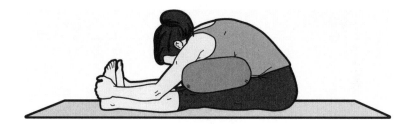

EQUIPMENT: bolster or rolled-up blanket

Sit on the floor with your spine long and your legs straight out in front of you.

Roll the tops of your thighs inward with your hands.

Fully extend your legs, pressing actively through the heels.

Place a bolster or rolled-up blanket across your thighs.

Leading with your sternum and keeping your torso long, move from your hip joints, extend forward, and hold the sides of either your feet or your shins.

Place your forehead on the bolster or blanket; adjust for comfort.

With each inhalation let your chest lift slightly; with each exhalation let your body relax deeply into the pose.

Release into the pose for 1 to 3 minutes.

SEATED UPRIGHT WIDE-ANGLE POSE
UPAVISTHA KONASANA

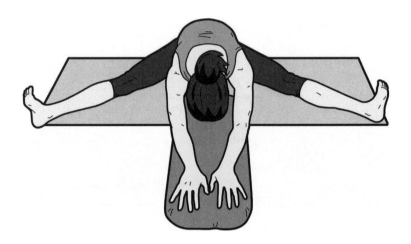

EQUIPMENT (OPTIONAL): 2 yoga blocks, folded blanket

Sit on the floor with your legs straight out in front of you.

Separate your legs to an angle of about 90 degrees.

Press your hands onto the floor and lift your pelvis to slide it
slightly forward, widening your legs another 10 to 20 degrees.

Press your thighs in toward the floor and rotate them outward, so
that your knees face straight up.

Lengthen your torso as you press though the balls of your feet.

Keep your hands pressing in front of you on the floor or yoga
blocks to keep your torso upright.

OPTIONAL: Place a folded blanket under your hips if it is difficult for
you to sit comfortably on the floor.

SEATED FORWARD WIDE-ANGLE POSE
UPAVISTHA KONASANA

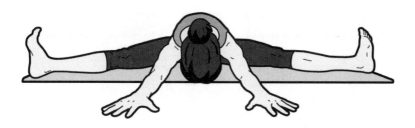

EQUIPMENT (OPTIONAL): bolster, blanket

Sit on the floor with your legs straight out in front of you.

Separate your legs to an angle of about 90 degrees.

Press your hands onto the floor and lift your pelvis to slide it slightly forward, widening the legs another 10 to 20 degrees.

Press your thighs in toward the floor and rotate them outward, so that the knees face straight up.

Lengthen your torso as you press though the balls of your feet.

Move from your hip joints, maintaining a long spine, as you lean forward onto a bolster, a rolled-up blanket, or the floor.

With each breath go deeper into the pose, maintaining length in your torso.

Start with five to ten breaths and work your way up to 1 to 3 minutes.

OPTIONAL: Place a folded blanket under your hips if it is difficult for you to sit comfortably on the floor.

SEATED LATERAL WIDE-ANGLE POSE
PARSVA UPAVISTHA KONASANA

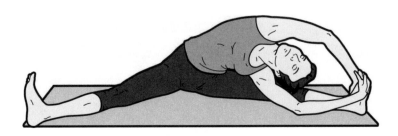

EQUIPMENT (OPTIONAL): bolster, blanket

Sit on the floor with your legs straight out in front of you.

Separate your legs to an angle of about 90 degrees.

Press your hands onto the floor and lift your pelvis to slide it slightly forward, widening your legs another 10 to 20 degrees.

Press your thighs in toward the floor and rotate them outward, so that your knees face straight up.

Lengthen your torso as you press though the balls of your feet.

Rotate your torso to the right.

Press your hands to either side of your right thigh.

Anchor your left hip and thigh on the floor.

Walk your hands down the leg, moving toward clasping your foot with your hands.

Place your head on a bolster, a rolled-up blanket, or your shin.

Keep anchoring your left hip and thigh down and maintaining length in both sides of the waist.

Stay for 1 minute, return to the upright position, switch sides, and repeat.

OPTIONAL: Place a folded blanket under your hips if it is difficult for you to sit comfortably on the floor.

SEATED REVOLVED WIDE-ANGLE POSE
PARIVRTTA UPAVISTHA KONASANA

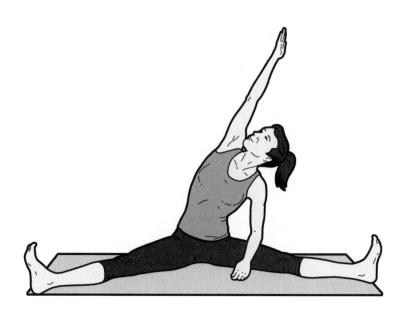

EQUIPMENT (OPTIONAL): blanket

Sit on the floor with your legs straight out in front of you.

Separate your legs to an angle of about 90 degrees.

Press your hands onto the floor and lift your pelvis to slide it slightly forward, widening your legs another 10 to 20 degrees.

Press your thighs in toward the floor and rotate them outward, so that your knees face straight up.

Lengthen your torso as you press though the balls of your feet.

Anchor your left hip and thigh on the floor as you place your right forearm on your right thigh.

Lean toward the right, extending your left arm toward the ceiling.

Maintain length in both sides of your torso as you turn slightly to the ceiling.

Stay for 1 minute, return to the upright position, and switch sides.

TO GO DEEPER: Place your right arm in front of your right thigh and reach your left arm overhead to clasp your left foot.

OPTIONAL: Place a folded blanket under your hips if it is difficult for you to sit comfortably on the floor.

BRIDGE POSE
SETU BANDA SARVANGASANA

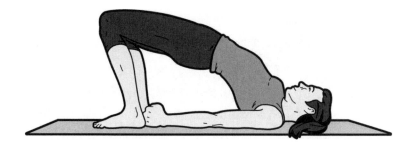

Lie on your back with your knees bent and your feet flat on the floor with your heels close to your pelvis.

Lengthen your neck, roll your shoulders back, and let your sternum gently lift up.

Press into your inner heels as you raise your pelvis off the floor.

Roll your shoulders into the floor again, lacing your hands beneath you on the mat.

Lengthen your tailbone toward the back of your knees, maintaining length in your spine.

Keep drawing your tailbone away from you as you press your feet down. Notice the rebound effect of receiving energy as you press into the floor with your feet and the back of your shoulders.

Remain in the pose for ten breaths, observing how each inhale extends the pose and each exhale takes you deeper within.

SUPPORTED BRIDGE POSE
SETU BANDA SARVANGASANA

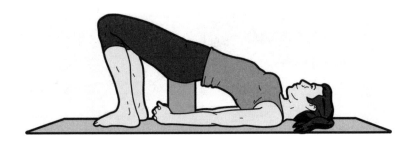

EQUIPMENT: yoga block or bolster

Lie on your back with your knees bent and your feet flat on the floor with your heels close to your pelvis.

Roll your shoulders back and lengthen your neck on the mat.

Exhale and press your feet down as you raise your pelvis off the floor.

Slide a yoga block, positioned the tall and narrow way, under your sacrum.

Lengthen your tailbone toward the back of your knees, maintaining length in your spine.

Let your thighs descend toward the floor.

Lace your hands beneath your back (or keep your arms at your sides), and keep your chest gently lifting.

Start with a few breaths and work your way up to 3 to 5 minutes.

OPTIONAL: If using a block is too difficult, use a shorter block or a bolster.

SUPPORTED GODDESS POSE
SUPTA BADDHA KONASANA

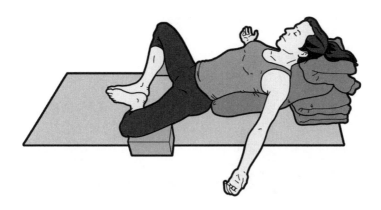

EQUIPMENT: 2 yoga blocks or a rolled-up blanket; bolster and folded blanket

Sit on the floor and bend your knees, bringing the soles of your feet together and letting your knees fall out to either side.

Place a rolled-up blanket or yoga block beneath each thigh and a bolster and folded blanket behind you.

Exhale and lean back onto the bolster with your head supported by the folded blanket.

Rotate your thighs gently outward.

Roll your shoulders gently down your back, lengthen the back of your neck, and release your arms to either side of you with your palms up.

Start with 1 to 2 minutes in this pose, working your way up to 5 to 10 minutes.

OPTIONAL: If this pose is challenging, sit cross-legged and/or use two bolsters instead of one.

LEGS UP THE WALL POSE
VIPARITA KARANI

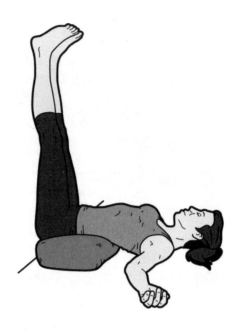

EQUIPMENT: 2 folded blankets or a bolster

Place two folded blankets or a bolster the long way in front of a wall, leaving about a hand's length between the bolster and the wall.

Sit sideways on the end of the bolster.

Exhale and swing your legs up onto the wall as you lower your torso to the floor.

Let your hips release into the space between the bolster and the wall.

Roll your shoulder blades down away from your neck and release your hands and arms out to your sides, palms up.

Start off for a few minutes in the pose and work your way up to 10 to 15 minutes.

To come out of the pose, slowly slide off the bolster onto the floor and stay flat on the floor for a few breaths before rolling onto your side to sit up.

NOTE: Viparita Karani is a wonderful therapeutic pose to practice but sometimes can be a challenge to learn how to get into. Adjust this pose according to your needs. If you are less flexible, use a lower height of blanket, and if you are petite, try moving the bolster closer to the wall. Discover what is most comfortable for you.

SUPPORTED CORPSE POSE
SAVASANA

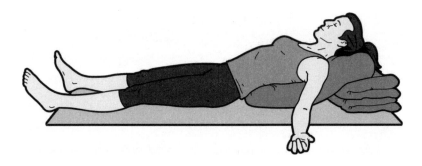

EQUIPMENT: bolster and a few folded blankets

Lie on the mat with your knees bent, supporting your upper back and head so that your heart and head are elevated.

Lift your hips up and roll your pelvis away from your back to extend your lower back.

Straighten one leg at a time on the floor, letting your feet turn out both evenly and comfortably.

Let your chest open and body relax.

Remain in the pose for 5 to 10 minutes.

To come out of the pose, roll to your side and remain there for a few breaths before sitting up.

SEATED POSE

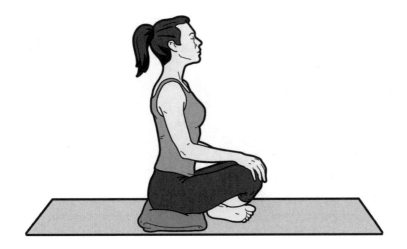

EQUIPMENT (OPTIONAL): folded blanket

Sit on the floor or on a folded blanket with your legs crossed comfortably.

Ground your hips evenly as you lengthen your spine.

Place your hands on your knees and lift through the chest.

Remain for five to ten breaths, then switch your crossed legs.

GENTLE TWIST

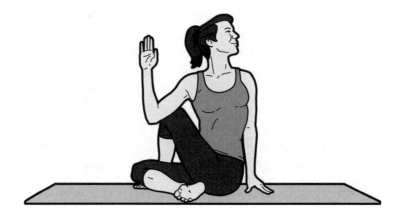

Sit on the floor with your legs extended.

Bend your knees, and place your left foot under your right leg and the right foot over the left leg with the right foot pressing actively on the floor and the right knee pointing toward the ceiling.

Lengthen your spine and twist as you press your right hand on the mat just behind your sacrum, and place your left arm on the outside of your right thigh.

Gently twist toward the right.

Continue to lengthen your spine with each breath.

Remain for five breaths and switch sides.

SEATED OVERHEAD EXTENSION

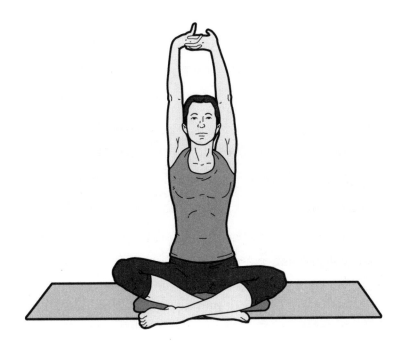

Sit cross-legged on your mat with your legs crossed comfortably.

Extend the arms over the head and lace your hands together, interlocking the fingers.

Turn your palms toward the sky, keeping your hands laced together.

Remain for five to ten breaths, then switch your crossed legs and interlocked fingers.

CHILD'S POSE

BALASANA

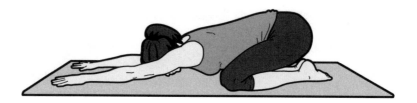

Go onto your hands and knees on the floor.

Place your big toes together and widen your knees.

Exhale and reach back with your hips as you lengthen your torso.

Place your torso down as your head comes to the floor.

Lengthen your tailbone away from your back as you extend your arms on the floor.

Let each inhale extend the spine and each exhale bring you deeper into the pose.

Start with a few breaths and work your way up to 5 minutes.

CHILD'S POSE WITH TRACTION

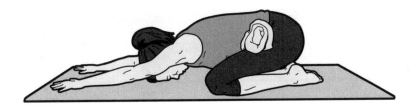

EQUIPMENT: rolled-up blanket

Kneel on the floor. Place your big toes together and widen your knees.

Place a rolled-up blanket in the fold of your hips.

Exhale and reach forward, drawing your belly over the blanket.

Walk your hands forward and extend your arms on the floor.

Allow the blanket to draw your hips back as you continue to stretch forward.

With each inhale, allow your torso to lift a bit, extending the spine. Then, with each exhale, fold deeper into the pose.

Start with a few breaths and work your way up to 5 minutes.

CORPSE POSE
SAVASANA

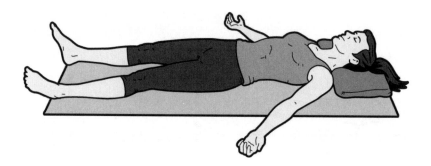

Lie on the floor with your knees bent and feet on the floor.

Lift your hips up and draw your hips gently toward your ribs to lengthen your lower back, then place your hips back down.

Straighten one leg at a time on the floor, letting your feet turn out both evenly and comfortably.

Gently roll your shoulders down your back, allowing the floor to provide traction. Relax your arms at your sides with your palms up.

Lengthen the back of your neck and close your eyes.

Soften into the pose.

Stay in Savasana for 5 to 15 minutes, then roll onto your side, staying in this transitional pose for a few breaths before using your arms to lift yourself up to sit.

———

If you want to go deeper in your yoga practice, you might want to check Wini's yoga and fitness programs on her Web site, www.bodychange .com.

I often tell my patients that true beauty is radiant health. This starts with the foods you eat. In fact, I have discovered that the greatest gift I can give my readers is permission to eat healthful food. In chapter 8, "The Forever Young Kitchen and Recipes," you will find food lists that are your best Forever Young choices as well as superb recipes from the wonderful people at Williams-Sonoma and B&W Quality Growers, growers of watercress and arugula.

Chapter Eight

THE FOREVER YOUNG KITCHEN AND RECIPES

Learning how to look and feel Forever Young starts with the foods you eat. This means that the kitchen takes on new importance, becoming perhaps the most important room in your home.

In this chapter we are going to share a selection of truly delicious recipes from two very special sources. The selection of recipes featuring watercress is courtesy of the Burgoon family, the owners of B&W Quality Growers introduced in chapter 4. I would like to thank the entire Burgoon family, including Dick, the owner, and his lovely wife, Pat, as well as Andy Brown, Dick's son-in-law and VP of marketing, for so generously sharing these outstanding recipes and the many amazing health benefits of watercress. If there is a fountain of youth, it may very well be found in a handful of foods—topping the list are surely watercress, wild salmon, and the remarkable chia seed!

A wonderful selection of recipes is also courtesy of *Williams-Sonoma Healthy Main Dishes,* a part of its New Healthy Kitchen Series, available at both www.barnesandnoble.com and www.amazon.com. What I treasure about this book is the focus on what I call the "rainbow foods," a concept I introduced in *The Perricone Promise* (Warner Books, 2003) and still believe in today—more than ever. Williams-Sonoma has the finest selection of just about everything related to the kitchen and fine cooking and dining—including its cookbooks. These books are a visual delight, and the recipes are sublime. I must have close to a dozen Williams-Sonoma cookbooks, so I can attest to that!

Salmon:
The World's Best Forever Young Secret

Not too long ago, Madonna, the ageless superstar, announced to the world that she was embarking on a "salmon rejuvenation" program to "knock twelve years off of her appearance."

Though it might be ambitious to think we can knock more than a decade off our looks, think again. If *anything* can do it, it is the anti-inflammatory lifestyle of diet, nutritional supplements, and topicals. This is because inflammation is responsible for many of the internal *and* external signs of aging.

Madonna's truly inspiring sense of determination and commitment will go a long way to helping her achieve her goals. Madonna's dedication to the salmon diet has also inspired me to have a little fun, as you will discover in the upcoming pages.

Why Eating Salmon Is Antiaging

I have to say it once more: I am probably the single greatest advocate for adding wild salmon and other omega-3 cold-water fish (think sardines, anchovies, halibut, sablefish, trout, and so on) to your daily diet.

Wild salmon contains essential fats and powerful antioxidants, such as the carotenoid astaxanthin, that have important anti-inflammatory properties.

Salmon is also probably the world's most heart-healthy source of protein. It is rich in long-chain omega-3 essential fatty acids—the most beneficial kind—which protect heart health, inhibit inflammation, act as natural antidepressants, increase feelings of well-being, and help keep skin young, supple, and radiant.

Protein for Cellular Repair

Wild salmon and other cold-water fish are great sources of protein, which is necessary to maintain and repair the body—including the skin—on a cellular level. The lack of protein is first visible in the face, even in a young person, but *especially as we age.*

Like a Surgeon

Not only plastic surgery can give you that sculpted look. Adequate protein is vital, because without protein, you will lose contours and definition in your face. This is another reason why a diet rich in salmon is important for Madonna if she wants to maintain that chiseled look of high cheekbones, well-defined jawline, good eye contours, and so on.

Protein cannot be stored in our bodies. For good health and outstanding cellular repair, protein needs to be eaten with each meal, and salmon is an outstanding protein source. Women, however, are very often protein-deficient, which shows up in their faces. Men, on the other hand, do tend to gravitate toward protein and are more likely to go for a burger or a steak while women choose a salad—or worse, a cookie. This is one reason (but not the only one) why men appear to age better than women.

Secret

As a dermatologist, I know that when it comes to their skin, women will invest great sums in topical products, procedures, and so forth. If it is the right product, with high, efficacious levels of anti-inflammatory antioxidants, they will see beautiful and gratifying results.

But there is a little beauty secret that is worth its weight in gold. If women understood that eating a simple, inexpensive small can of sardines or salmon would give their skin an unrivaled radiance, softness, and suppleness, like *nothing else in this world,* those foods would fly off the supermarket shelves. You would see a *stampede* toward the fish aisle. While the extraordinary multiorgan benefits of sardines and wild salmon almost sound like a fantasy, they are very real. Try canned salmon and sardines, which also contain both skin and bones, to experience just a few of these skin, brain, mood, and health and energy benefits of these amazing omega-3-, protein-, and calcium-rich fish, including:

- Decreased inflammation in all organ systems, including the skin
- Decreased body fat
- Ample quantities of high-quality fat and protein
- Beautiful skin
- Elevated mood
- Improved brain function
- Increased energy
- Improved athletic ability
- Decreased puffiness
- Decreased fine lines and wrinkles
- Decreased sagging
- Increased radiance and glow
- Dramatically improved acne and decreased acne scarring
- Improved attention span
- Stabilized blood sugar levels
- Lowered insulin levels
- Healthy serotonin levels
- Decreased appetite

- Healthier immune system
- Increased energy levels
- Decreased symptoms and severity of rheumatoid arthritis
- Reduced symptoms and severity of chronic skin conditions such as eczema
- Decreased stroke and cardiovascular risk
- Decreased pain and inflammation in joints

With a list of benefits like this, how can you resist?

Beautiful Stranger

I am guardedly optimistic that Madonna, ever the trendsetter, will inspire women everywhere to try the "salmon rejuvenation" program.

To be Forever Young—or to at least look and feel your finest—follow the anti-inflammatory diet, which consists of the following:

- High-quality protein, like that found in fish, shellfish, poultry, and tofu
- Low-glycemic carbohydrates (these will not provoke a glycemic response when consumed in moderation), including

HARD CANDY BLUES

Avoiding sugary, starchy foods is also essential, as these types of foods blur our contours, giving our faces a soft, doughy look. In fact, it is always easy to spot people who are addicted to these types of carbs because they do not have attractive facial contours.

colorful fresh fruits and vegetables, whole grains such as old-fashioned oatmeal, and legumes such as beans and lentils
- Healthy fats, such as those found in cold-water fish (especially wild salmon, halibut, sardines, herring, anchovies, and trout), nuts, seeds, and olive oil
- Eight to ten glasses of pure spring water per day
- Antioxidant-rich beverages, such as green tea

You will notice a visible difference in as little as three days, with even more dramatic results by week's end. After four weeks, your friends and family will be commenting on how different you look.

And when you look in the mirror, you may begin to wonder, "Who's that girl?"

Salmon: Fish for Compliments
Anti-inflammatory Extraordinaire

If we are going to rate a food group as either pro-inflammatory or anti-inflammatory, we will find that protein, on the whole, is neutral. However, some sources of protein, such as the fish listed above, provide powerful anti-inflammatory benefits because of two of their constituents:

- Omega-3 essential fatty acids
- The carotenoid antioxidant astaxanthin, introduced in chapter 4

Thus wild salmon is anti-inflammatory. Beef and other forms of meat that are not grass-fed, like most meat available in supermarkets, tend to be high in saturated fats, making them pro-inflammatory.

The Borderline:
Moderation Is Key

Madonna has also reportedly started a more cardiointensive gym routine. Her rigorous routines are already legendary. But she needs to be careful and not subject her body to too extreme a workout. She should exercise some restraint because overexercising can produce inflammation-generating free radicals. It is not just pollution, poor diet, and the like that generate an abundance of free radicals; they also result from the metabolic process that takes place internally from overexercising and can damage the cell's DNA. That is why the previous chapter is dedicated to yoga. Madonna (surprise!) is reportedly an avid practitioner of Ashtanga yoga, a particularly strenuous form.

Exercise is vital to your health. It is also unsurpassed at lowering blood sugar, a key antiaging strategy. There are many studies proving that exercise can take off pounds, reduce the incidence of heart disease, lower blood pressure, improve mood, solve sleep problems, and even cut the risks of certain cancers. Exercise will also ensure that you have beautiful skin. Studies have indicated that exercise benefits the skin in much the same way it improves bone and muscle quality.

Youthful Skin—Naturally

When the skin of those who exercise regularly is examined under a microscope, the impact of their high fitness levels is clearly apparent. The skin is thicker and has more and healthier collagen, the fibers that give the skin its strength and flexibility. Exercise also increases circulation and gives the skin a healthy, radiant glow.

Bedtime Stories

Having an exciting romantic life is also a key to looking younger than our years. With the press reporting on Madonna's active love life with

MORE LOVE AT FIRST BITE:
FOODS TO HELP RENEW THE LIBIDO

No, this section is not about the HBO hit series *True Blood*. And you won't find one mention of vampires, Bon Temps, Louisiana, Anna Paquin, or Stephen Moyer. What you will discover is the anti-inflammatory diet (not a drop of synthetic blood on the menu), which will work wonders for your sex life. As we have seen, chocolate has many benefits, including its ability to mimic the sensation of being in love. In addition to chocolate, here is a selection of foods that can help increase the libido and promote the loss of unwanted body fat, which will help make you feel more attractive—always a boost when it comes to the libido.

Healthy fats are vital to hormone production, and a healthy sex life is all about the hormones. Here is a short list of some wonderful foods that will go a long way toward enhancing your sex life as well as your overall sense of happiness.

1. Wild salmon and other cold-water fish (sardines, herring, trout, and anchovies, to name a few) are high in omega-3 fats. In fact, if you want just *one* food group that is guaranteed to help increase overall health and sexual stamina, these fish are for you. Omega-3s are critical to the brain and nervous system. They also improve your mood, increase your sense of well-being, fight depression, give you glowing, radiant skin, and improve your memory and brain-power.

2. Watermelon is rich in L-citrulline, an amino acid that helps improve blood flow. L-citrulline supports the body in optimizing blood flow when it converts to L-arginine and then to nitric oxide. Nitric oxide is involved in vasodilation (dilation of the blood vessels). Low levels of nitric oxide are associated with mental and physical fatigue and sexual dysfunction. Like Viagra, L-citrulline increases blood flow to the sexual organs but without any negative side effects. In fact, some experts are asking, "Is watermelon the new Viagra?"

3. Extra-dark chocolate contains phenylethylamine, a chemical believed to produce the feeling of being in love. We all know how good chocolate makes us feel. In fact, a study published in *The Journal of Sexual Medicine* found that women who enjoyed a piece of chocolate every day had a more active sex life than those who didn't.

4. Asparagus is rich in folate, a B vitamin that helps increase the production of histamine. The correct levels of histamine are important for a healthy sex drive in both men and women.

5. Oysters are extremely rich in zinc, essential for testosterone production and the maintenance of healthy sperm. And even though women have much less testosterone than men, it also plays a key part in the female libido. Oysters also boost dopamine, a hormone that increases libido in both men and women.

6. Blueberries. When it comes to boosting dopamine levels, blueberries rule. Blueberries give the body a greater ability to release dopamine, an energizing, stimulatory neurotransmitter. They also protect us from the loss of dopamine cells normally seen with aging. By increasing brain energy production and maintaining youthful brain function, dopamine exerts an extremely important antiaging effect. Since dopamine levels decrease with age, blueberries become even more important as we get older.

7. Pumpkin seeds. Pumpkin seeds, like oysters, are extremely rich in zinc and promote the health of the male prostate gland. And don't underestimate the power of zinc when it comes to a woman's sex drive. One study found that pumpkin seeds are a great libido booster. Pumpkin seeds are rich in omega-3 essential fatty acids, which act as a precursor of prostaglandins—hormonelike substances important for sexual health.

8. Garlic contains allicin, a compound thought to increase blood flow to the sexual organs. Some experts believe that garlic is a very powerful aphrodisiac. But garlic doesn't work overnight. It is necessary to take capsules or eat garlic daily for about a month to reap its remarkable benefits.

9. Avocado is rich in folic acid for increased energy production and healthy fats to improve mood and sense of well-being.

10. Peanuts, especially for men. Studies show that the amino acid L-arginine is helpful for improving sexual function in men. L-arginine is used to make nitric oxide, which relaxes blood vessels. Preliminary studies have found that L-arginine may help with erectile dysfunction because it relaxes the blood vessels. Peanuts are a rich natural source of L-arginine.

---

a series of younger, handsome, and extremely fit men, we can again be assured that she is leaving no stone unturned in her quest for the fountain of youth.

Enjoying a healthy and robust sexuality confers many health and longevity benefits. Some studies even suggest that sexual activity may be associated with reducing the risk of the two leading causes of death in the United States: heart disease and cancer.

Lucky Star

We wish Madonna much luck on her salmon regimen. Her hard work and self-discipline have kept her at the top for more than two decades. Though I can't promise that she can turn back time, the anti-inflammatory benefits of foods such as salmon will guarantee that she can greatly slow down its negative effects while emphasizing the positive. These include good health, ample energy, increased sense of well-being, and radiant, glowing skin.

In other words, we can be sure that she will live to tell us all about it, in her own inimitable way.

A Note on Chia Seeds

As you have read throughout this book, chia seeds are truly a superfood for their many benefits: healthy weight loss, their omega-3 profile, and their considerable (and unique) ability to increase endurance and stamina. I want to again thank Bob Terry, Ph.D., the technical service adviser of Green Foods Corporation, for his outstanding scientific insights and Jason Nava, the executive vice president of Green Foods Corporation, for generous help in explaining the benefits of both chia seeds and the green foods.

The Best Foods to Choose When Stocking the Forever Young Kitchen

Fish and Seafood

According to the Environmental Defense Fund (www.edf.org), the following fish are the eco-best choices.

Abalone	Lobster, Caribbean spiny, U.S.
Anchovies (European)	Mahimahi, U.S. troll/pole
Bass, striped, farmed	Mullet
Clams, farmed	Mussels
Clams, soft-shell	Oysters, farmed
Crawfish, U.S.	Prawns, Canada
Cod, Alaskan, longline	Sablefish/black cod, Alaska
Halibut, Pacific	Salmon, canned
Lobster, Cabaja spiny	Salmon, wild

Sardines, Pacific, U.S.
Scallops, bay, farmed
Shrimp, Oregon

Squid, longfin, U.S.
Tilapia, U.S.
Trout, farmed

Meat and Poultry

Beef, 100% grass-fed
Chicken and turkey, free-range,
    raised without added hor-
    mones and antibiotics, never
    fed animal by-products

Lamb, 100% grass-fed

Dairy Products

Choose organic, low fat (unless from grass-fed animals) including:

Butter (use in moderation)
Buttermilk
Cheese (especially Parmigiano-
    Reggiano and sheep and goat
    milk cheeses such as feta,
    Pecorino Romano, etc.)
Cheese, cottage

Cheese, farmer
Eggs, organic, from free-range
    chickens
Kefir
Milk
Ricotta
Yogurt

Healthy Fats

Coconut oil, virgin
Olive oil—extra-virgin olive oil is
    the recommended variety

Olives, black and green

Whole Grains

Barley
Oatmeal, slow-cooking

Oats, whole or steel cut

Nuts and Seeds

Almonds

Almond butter

Brazil nuts

Chestnuts

Chia seeds (see page 265)

Hazelnuts

Macadamia nuts

Peanuts

Peanut butter, old-fashioned
(avoid commercial peanut
butter)

Pecans

Pine nuts

Pistachios

Pumpkin seeds

Sesame seeds

Sesame tahini

Sunflower seeds

Walnuts

Fruits and Vegetables

NOTE: Save sweet fresh fruit for the end of the meal to keep your blood
sugar levels normal.

Apples

Artichokes

Arugula

Asparagus

Bamboo shoots

Berries (blackberries, blueberries,
raspberries, strawberries, etc.)

Bok choy

Broccoli

Broccoli rabe

Cabbage

Cantaloupe

Cauliflower

Celeriac (celery root)

Chard, Swiss

Cherries

Chestnuts, water

Chicory

Chinese cabbage

Collards

Cucumbers

Dandelion greens

Eggplant

Endive

Escarole

Garlic

Grapefruit

Kale

Kohlrabi

Leeks

Lemons

Lentils

Lettuce, dark red and dark green
varieties

Lettuce, romaine

Limes

Melon, honeydew

Mushrooms

Muskmelon

Natto (fermented soy product
high in bone-building vitamin K2)

Onions

Oranges (temple, mandarin,
blood, navel, etc.)

Parsley

Pea pods

Peas, snow

Pears

Peppers, green, red, yellow, and
orange bell

Peppers, hot (cherry, serrano,
jalapeño, etc.)

Pineapple

Plums

Pomegranates

Potatoes, sweet

Quinoa

Radicchio

Radish, daikon

Radishes

Rhubarb

Rutabagas

Scallions

Sea vegetables (nori, kelp, arame,
dulse, etc.)

Shallots

Soba (buckwheat noodles)

Sorrel

Spinach

Sprouts

Sprouts, bean

Sprouts, broccoli

Sprouts, brussels

Squash

Squash, summer

Squash, winter

String beans

Tangelos

Tangerines

Tofu

Tomatoes

Turnips

Watercress

Watermelon

Zucchini

Herbs and Spices

Allspice

Anise

Basil

Bay leaf

Black pepper

Capers

Caraway seed

Cardamom

Cayenne pepper

Celery seed

Chervil

Chili powder

Chives

Cilantro

Cinnamon

Cloves

Coriander

Cumin

Dill

Fennel

Gingerroot

Marjoram

Mint

Mustard

Nutmeg

Oregano

Paprika

Parsley

Red pepper flakes

Rosemary

Tarragon

Thyme

Turmeric

Saffron

Sage

Savory

Vanilla beans

Beans and Legumes, Dried and Fresh

Beans, adzuki

Beans, Anasazi

Beans, Appaloosa

Beans, black

Beans, calypso

Beans, cannellini

Beans, cranberry

Beans, European soldier

Beans, fava

Beans, flageolet

Beans, great northern

Beans, lima (butter)

Beans, lupini

Beans, mung

Beans, pinto

Beans, red

Beans, red kidney

Beans, trout

Chickpeas

Lentils (all varieties)

Peas, black-eyed

Peas, green

Peas, split

Beverages

Tea, green

Note on Cookware

Many recipes call for nonstick cookware, but the jury is out on this topic. I recommend Le Creuset. Le Creuset is the world's leading manufacturer of enameled cast-iron cookware that is as beautiful as it is functional. The only challenge when it comes to shopping for Le Creuset is choosing the color! All Le Creuset cookware is made from enameled cast iron. Cast iron has been used for cooking utensils since the Middle Ages. The Le Creuset factory is located in Fresnoy-le-Grand in northern France. Since much of the finishing is done by hand, each Le Creuset cast-iron cookware piece is completely unique.

For elegant yet practical selections of the finest dinnerware, chef's tools, linens, recipes, cookware, and more, visit www.williams-sonoma.com.

A Note on Dried Beans

Since cooked dried beans take so well to a variety of seasonings, chefs love to experiment with them. In addition, beans are an excellent source of resistant starch (RS). These fiberlike carbohydrates are the unsung heroes of weight control. They increase the rate at which the body burns (oxidizes) body fat, do not cause unhealthy spikes in blood sugar levels, and prevent other, higher-glycemic foods in a meal from doing so.

The benefits of eating foods high in RS are as follows.

- Resistant starch resists digestion and absorption as it passes through the small intestine, where most dietary starch is digested. It then passes into the large intestine, where it behaves much like insoluble fiber, promoting the growth of beneficial bacteria and the production of disease-preventive fatty acids.
- RS is digested slowly, thereby preventing an inflammatory spike in blood sugar levels.

- When you eat a small amount of RS—for instance, a handful of beans or chickpeas—it will prevent higher-glycemic foods in the meal from causing inflammatory spikes in blood sugar and insulin levels.
- Because of its probiotic fermentation-enhancing effects in the digestive system, RS even improves long-term insulin sensitivity.
- Like omega-3s, RS possesses the unique ability to increase thermogenesis (the burning of body fat). One study found that those eating a meal containing a small amount of RS showed a 20 percent increase in thermogenesis that lasted for twenty-four hours.
- Beans contain phytonutrients called amylase inhibitors, which block the action of the enzyme amylase needed to digest starches. This effect should help prevent the digestion of some of the starch in the beans themselves, as well as the starch in other foods eaten with beans.

The only trick with beans is to cook them until they are tender. Crunch is not what you want from a bean. That said, to properly cook dried beans, first soak them one of two ways: either in very hot water for an hour or two at room temperature, or cover them with cold water and refrigerate overnight. The next step is to drain them, put them in a pot, cover by 2 inches with water, and simmer gently until tender. Then season as desired.

Recipes

Many of these recipes contain cruciferous and carotenoid vegetables. This is by careful design, as our goal is to protect all parts of the cell, especially the mitochondria and mitochondrial DNA, from damage. As we learned in chapter 1, cellular damage, particularly to the mitochondrial DNA, is responsible for cellular aging. In addition, cruciferous vegetables influence gene expression, as do cocoa, tea, berries, and many spices, including turmeric and cinnamon.

This means that these foods can actually block the damaging and age-accelerating transcription factors that promote disease and wrinkled, sagging skin while turning on the transcription factors that stop disease, keep all organ systems functioning at optimal levels, and maintain radiant and youthful skin. Since watercress is an outstanding example of these superfoods, we have included many wonderful recipes utilizing this miracle green.

Preparing and enjoying these delicious recipes will be a key strategy in keeping you Forever Young and Forever Healthy.

Bon appétit!

Appetizers

WATERCRESS AND BRIE-TOPPED ARTICHOKE HEARTS

Makes 18 pieces of delicious finger food

One 9-ounce box frozen artichoke hearts
⅔ cup finely chopped blanched watercress (see page 273),
    about 2 bunches, trimmed
1 teaspoon lemon pepper
¼ teaspoon salt
18 thin slices Brie cheese

1. Preheat the broiler.
2. Cook the artichoke hearts, following the package directions, and drain them well.

3. Combine the watercress, lemon pepper, and salt in a small bowl.

4. Place the artichoke hearts on a baking sheet, and top each one with a portion of the watercress mixture. Lay the Brie on top, and broil until the cheese melts, 1 to 2 minutes.

WATERCRESS DIP WITH CHIPOTLE AND LIME

Serve this dip with a selection of fresh raw vegetables, such as broccoli and cauliflower florets, carrot sticks, and celery sticks.

Makes 3 cups

5 bunches or bags B&W watercress, trimmed
8 ounces cream cheese (about 1 cup), at room temperature
1 cup plain yogurt
½ cup chopped scallions
⅓ cup fresh cilantro
1 tablespoon chopped chipotle in adobo sauce, or more to taste
1 tablespoon sea salt, or to taste
Freshly ground black pepper

1. Bring a large saucepan of water to a boil. Have ready a large bowl of ice water.

2. Blanch the watercress in the boiling water for 1 to 1½ minutes until just tender. Drain, and immediately submerge the watercress in the ice water. When the watercress has cooled, drain it well and bundle it in a clean dish towel. Squeeze it very tightly to extract all excess moisture. Set aside.

3. Combine the cream cheese and all the remaining ingredients in a food processor, and blend until very smooth, about 90 seconds. Add the watercress and pulse until just combined. Taste, and adjust the seasoning if necessary.

PUREED LENTILS*

Serve this as a dip with an assortment of crisp raw vegetables, such as broccoli florets, celery sticks, and carrot sticks.

2 cups dried lentils
1 tablespoon olive oil
½ red bell pepper, roasted, peeled, and coarsely chopped
Sea salt and freshly ground black pepper

1. Bring a pot of salted water to a boil. Add the lentils, reduce the heat, and simmer, covered, until soft, about 20 minutes. Drain well.
2. Transfer the lentils to a food processor or blender, and add the olive oil, bell pepper, and sea salt and black pepper to taste; puree.

* This recipe, and others starred, comes from *Williams-Sonoma New Healthy Kitchen: Main Dishes.* Copyright © 2006 by Weldon Owen. Reprinted by permission of Weldon Owen and Free Press, a Division of Simon & Schuster, Inc. All rights reserved.

Savory Soups

CHICKEN EGG DROP SOUP WITH WATERCRESS

Serves 4

6 cups low-sodium chicken broth
½ cup finely diced celery
2 tablespoons minced onion
2 large eggs, well beaten
2 bunches B&W watercress, trimmed

1. Bring the chicken broth to a boil in a large pot. Add the celery and onion and simmer, covered, until tender, about 10 minutes.

2. With the soup at a rapid boil, slowly pour in the beaten eggs, stirring until the eggs form fine shreds. Add the watercress and cook only about a minute longer.

COLD WATERCRESS AND AVOCADO SOUP

Serves 4

1 quart low-sodium chicken broth
2 bunches fresh watercress, trimmed and chopped
4 avocados, pitted, peeled, and sliced
4 stems fresh cilantro, chopped
2 cups plain yogurt
2 tablespoons crème fraîche
Salt and freshly ground black pepper, to taste
Juice of 2 limes
1 green chili, such as jalapeño, finely chopped (optional)

1. Bring the broth to a simmer in a large saucepan. Set aside a few watercress leaves for garnish, and then add the remaining watercress to the stock. Simmer for 15 minutes.
2. Strain the broth into a container and let cool to room temperature. Then refrigerate until thoroughly chilled.
3. Combine all the remaining ingredients in a food processor and blend until smooth. Taste, and adjust the seasoning if necessary. Cover and refrigerate until thoroughly chilled.
4. To serve, stir the creamy avocado mixture into the broth, and garnish with the reserved watercress leaves.

CREAMY ARTICHOKE AND WATERCRESS SOUP

Pureed artichoke hearts, in addition to eggs, thicken this delectable version of the classic Greek soup avgolemono. Watercress adds extra color and nutrients to the traditional lemony broth and rice.

Serves 2

Two 14-ounce cans reduced-sodium chicken broth
¼ cup rice
One 14-ounce can artichoke hearts, drained and rinsed
2 large eggs, at room temperature
2 to 3 tablespoons fresh lemon juice, to taste
1½ tablespoons chopped fresh dill
4 cups packed (2 bunches or bags) B&W watercress:
    a few sprigs reserved for garnish, the remainder cut into
    2-inch pieces
⅛ teaspoon freshly ground black pepper

1. Combine the broth and rice in a large saucepan, and bring to a boil over high heat. Reduce the heat to a simmer and cook, uncovered, until the rice is very tender, about 15 minutes.
2. Place the artichoke hearts, eggs, and lemon juice in a blender and puree. With the machine running, ladle about half of the rice mixture through the opening in the cover, and puree until smooth. (Use caution when pureeing hot liquids.) Return the pureed mixture to the saucepan and cook, stirring constantly, until an instant-read thermometer registers 160°F, reducing the heat as necessary to prevent the soup from boiling.
3. Stir in the dill, watercress, and pepper. Garnish with the reserved sprigs of watercress.

ROAST TURKEY, WATERCRESS, AND WINTER VEGETABLE CHOWDER

Think of this recipe as a basic formula for improvising with fresh vegetables and seasonings that appeal to you. Toss in a couple of chopped garlic cloves, a handful of torn fresh basil leaves, and a pinch or two of red pepper flakes or a minced chili pepper along with the thyme. Or add a can of drained and rinsed cannellini beans. Be creative. Let your imagination wander. Turn a soup into a hearty meal!

Serves 8

3 slices turkey bacon, diced
1 large yellow onion, cut into ½-inch dice
2 large stalks celery, cut into ½-inch dice
1 small butternut squash (about 1 pound), peeled,
    halved lengthwise, seeded, and cut into ½-inch dice
7 cups low-sodium chicken broth
3 cups fresh watercress, cut into 3-inch lengths
2 cups diced roast turkey (½-inch dice)
1 medium zucchini, cut into ½-inch dice
2 tablespoons minced fresh flat-leaf parsley
1 tablespoon minced fresh thyme
Salt and freshly ground black pepper

1. In a heavy 6- to 8-quart saucepan, cook the bacon over medium heat, stirring frequently, until browned. Using a slotted spoon, transfer the bacon to a plate. Set aside.
2. Pour off all but 2 tablespoons of the bacon fat, and return the pot to medium heat. Add the onion and celery, and sauté until the vegetables are soft but not browned, 3 to 5 minutes.
3. Add the squash and the broth, and bring to a boil. Then reduce the heat to a simmer, partially cover the pot, and cook until the squash is tender, about 15 minutes.

4. Add the watercress, turkey, zucchini, parsley, thyme, and reserved bacon. Cook for 3 to 5 minutes.

5. Add salt and pepper to taste. Ladle the soup into warmed bowls or mugs to serve.

WATERCRESS AND CAULIFLOWER SOUP

Serves 6

1 tablespoon unsalted butter
1 small onion, coarsely chopped (about 1 cup)
1 small head cauliflower (about 1¾ pounds),
    cut into 1-inch florets
2 cups low-sodium chicken broth
2½ teaspoons coarse salt
Freshly ground black pepper
1 bunch fresh watercress, thick stems removed (about 5 cups),
    a few small sprigs reserved for garnish

1. Melt the butter in a medium saucepan over medium heat. Add the onion and cook, stirring occasionally, until soft and translucent, about 5 minutes.

2. Add the cauliflower, broth, salt, ¼ teaspoon pepper, and 2 cups water. Bring to a boil. Cover, reduce the heat to a simmer, and cook, stirring once, until the cauliflower is very tender, about 15 minutes.

3. Remove the pan from the heat, and stir in the watercress.

4. Working in batches, puree the soup in a blender, filling the container no more than halfway each time.

5. Return the soup to the saucepan; cover to keep warm.

6. To serve, divide among 6 bowls. Garnish each bowl with a sprig of watercress, and season with pepper.

Seafood Main Dishes

BRAISED COD WITH BOK CHOY

Serves 4

2 tablespoons low-sodium soy sauce, plus more for serving
2 tablespoons dry white wine
½ clove garlic, minced
1 teaspoon minced fresh ginger
1 head bok choy, trimmed and coarsely chopped
4 cod or other firm fish fillets, such as halibut (4 to 6 ounces each)

1. Stir the soy sauce, wine, garlic, and ginger together in a small bowl. Set aside.
2. Immerse the bok choy in a bowl of water. Lift it from the water, letting the excess water drain off, and transfer it to a large sauté pan. Place over medium-high heat, add ¼ cup water, cover, bring to a boil, then reduce the heat to low. Cook until tender, 4 to 5 minutes.
3. Pour off the liquid and return the pan to low heat. Stir in the soy sauce mixture. Place the fish fillets on top of the bok choy, cover, and cook until the fish is opaque throughout, about 4 minutes.
4. Serve with soy sauce.

HALIBUT WITH LEMON-GARLIC OIL
AND SAUTÉED WATERCRESS

Serves 4

¼ cup extra-virgin olive oil
2 garlic cloves: 1 crushed, 1 minced
Finely grated zest of 1 lemon
½ teaspoon anchovy paste
Pinch of crushed red pepper flakes

7 bunches fresh watercress, trimmed and coarsely chopped
Salt and freshly ground black pepper
Four 6-ounce skinless halibut fillets

1. Preheat the oven to 400°F.
2. In a small bowl, combine 2 tablespoons of the olive oil with the crushed garlic and the lemon zest. Let stand at room temperature for 10 minutes, and then discard the garlic.
3. Meanwhile, heat 1 tablespoon of the olive oil in a large skillet over medium heat. Add the minced garlic, anchovy paste, and crushed red pepper flakes and cook, stirring, until fragrant, about 30 seconds. Add the watercress, raise the heat to medium-high, and cook, stirring, until barely wilted, about 3 minutes. Season with salt and black pepper, and set aside.
4. Heat the remaining 1 tablespoon olive oil in a large ovenproof skillet over high heat until shimmering. Season the halibut fillets with salt and black pepper, and add them to the skillet. Cook until beginning to brown on the bottom, about 3 minutes. Transfer the skillet to the oven and roast the halibut for about 5 minutes, or until just white throughout.
5. Warm the watercress mixture over medium-high heat until hot but still crisp-tender, about 1 minute. Spoon the watercress onto plates. Using a spatula, transfer the halibut, browned side up, to the plates. Drizzle with the lemon-garlic oil and serve.

MUSTARD AND CORIANDER-CRUSTED SALMON WITH WATERCRESS

Serves 4

1 tablespoon coriander seeds
1 teaspoon mustard seeds
Pinch of crushed red pepper flakes

1¼ pounds skinless wild salmon fillet, in 1 piece

Salt and freshly ground black pepper

1 tablespoon plus ½ teaspoon Dijon mustard

1 tablespoon plus 1 teaspoon extra-virgin olive oil

1 tablespoon fresh lemon juice

2 bunches or bags B&W watercress (8 ounces),
   thick stems discarded

1 cup tightly packed fresh flat-leaf parsley leaves

1. Preheat the oven to 425°F.

2. Combine the coriander seeds, mustard seeds, and crushed red pepper flakes in a spice grinder, and coarsely grind.

3. Season the salmon fillet with salt and black pepper, and spread the 1 tablespoon mustard evenly over the fillet. Press the ground spices into the mustard.

4. Heat the 1 teaspoon oil in a large nonstick ovenproof skillet over high heat. Add the salmon fillet, mustard side down, and cook until lightly browned, 2 to 3 minutes. Carefully turn the salmon over, and transfer the skillet to the oven. Roast the salmon for 6 minutes, or until cooked through. Transfer the fillet to a cutting board.

5. Meanwhile, in a medium bowl, whisk the lemon juice with the remaining 1 tablespoon olive oil and ½ teaspoon mustard. Add the watercress and parsley, season with salt and black pepper, and toss to coat. Cut the salmon fillet into 4 pieces and serve with the salad.

SALMON FILLETS WITH PUY LENTILS*

Lentils, like other legumes, are low in fat and high in protein and fiber, but they have the added advantage of cooking quickly. Lentils have a mild, often earthy flavor, and they're best if cooked with assertive flavorings. The best, most delicate lentils are the peppery French green lentils called *lentilles du Puy*. These choice lentils were originally grown in the volcanic soils of Puy in France, but now they're also grown in North America and Italy. They're especially good in salads, since they remain firm after cooking and have a rich flavor. They cook a bit more slowly than other lentils.

Serves 4

1½ cups Puy lentils
1½ tablespoons olive oil
2 tablespoons minced shallots or yellow onion
Salt
4 skin-on salmon fillets (4 to 6 ounces each)
Freshly ground black pepper
1 cup arugula (my favorite) or mixed salad greens

1. Pick over the lentils, then rinse and drain them well.
2. Heat 1 tablespoon of the oil in a saucepan over high heat. Add the shallots and lentils, and cook, stirring, until the shallots are translucent and the lentils glisten, about 2 minutes.
3. Add 4 cups water and ½ teaspoon salt, and bring to a boil. Then reduce the heat to medium-low, cover, and simmer until the lentils are tender but firm and most of the water has been absorbed, 30 to 35 minutes.
4. Meanwhile, place a rack in the upper third of the oven and preheat the oven to 500°F. Lightly grease a baking dish that is just large enough to hold the salmon in a single layer.

5. Rub the salmon fillets on both sides with the remaining ½ tablespoon olive oil; season with salt and pepper. Place the fillets in the prepared baking dish and roast until the fish flakes easily with a fork and is still translucent only in the center, 13 to 15 minutes.

6. When the lentils are done, remove the pan from the heat and drain well. Return the lentil mixture to the pan. Taste, and add salt if needed. Cover to keep warm.

7. To serve, divide the lentils among 4 plates and top each bed of lentils with a salmon fillet. Garnish with the arugula and serve at once.

SMOKED PAPRIKA-ROASTED SALMON WITH WILTED WATERCRESS

Serves 8

¼ cup fresh orange juice

2 tablespoons plus 1 teaspoon olive oil

2 teaspoons fresh thyme leaves

2 pounds wild salmon fillets

1 tablespoon mild smoked paprika

1 teaspoon Saigon cinnamon (available at most supermarkets)

1 teaspoon grated orange zest

½ teaspoon sea salt

3 bunches B&W watercress

1. Mix the orange juice, the 2 tablespoons oil, and 1 teaspoon of the thyme in a small bowl. Place the salmon in large glass baking dish, add the marinade, and turn to coat well. Cover and refrigerate for 30 minutes.

2. Preheat the oven to 400°F. Line a baking dish with foil, and grease the foil.

3. Mix the paprika, cinnamon, orange zest, sea salt, and remaining 1 teaspoon thyme in a small bowl.

4. Remove the salmon from the marinade and place it in the prepared baking dish; discard any remaining marinade. Rub the smoked paprika mixture evenly over the salmon. Roast in the oven for 10 to 15 minutes, or until the fish flakes easily with a fork.

5. Wash and trim the watercress. Heat the remaining teaspoon oil, add the watercress, and cook, stirring, for 2 minutes or until wilted. Serve the salmon over the watercress.

GRILLED TROUT WITH GOLDEN SQUASH KABOBS*

Serves 4

8 sunburst squash or yellow zucchini, cut into 1-inch chunks
2 teaspoons minced fresh thyme
2 tablespoons olive oil
½ teaspoon freshly ground black pepper
2 slices preservative-free bacon or turkey bacon,
    cut into ½-inch pieces (optional)
4 to 8 skin-on trout fillets (3 to 6 ounces each)

1. Toss the squash, thyme, 1 tablespoon of the oil, and the pepper together in a bowl. Let marinate for about 45 minutes, tossing occasionally.

2. Meanwhile, soak 4 long or 8 short wooden skewers in water for 30 minutes. Build a hot wood or charcoal fire in a grill, or preheat a gas grill to 400°F.

3. Thread the squash, alternating with the bacon if using, onto the soaked skewers. Grill until the squash is lightly browned and the bacon is beginning to crisp, 3 to 4 minutes per side. Transfer the skewers to a platter.

4. Brush the trout fillets with the remaining 1 tablespoon oil and place them, skin side down, on the grill. Cover the grill and cook until the fish is opaque throughout, 4 to 5 minutes. Transfer to a platter.

5. To serve, arrange 1 or 2 fillets on each plate and top with a kabob or two. (Or, remove the squash and bacon from the skewers, mound on each plate, and top with the fish.)

Main-Course Seafood Salads

KING CRAB AND WATERCRESS SALAD

Serves 4

4 bunches or bags B&W watercress, large stems trimmed
4 cooked Alaskan king crab legs, shelled, cartilage removed, meat cut into 3-inch pieces and chilled
16 cherry tomatoes
16 small mozzarella balls
½ avocado, pitted and peeled
Extra-virgin olive oil
Aged balsamic vinegar
Sea salt and freshly ground black pepper

1. Divide the watercress and crabmeat among 4 large soup plates, and arrange the tomatoes and mozzarella balls attractively around the watercress. Thinly slice the avocado and add it to the plates.

2. Drizzle with olive oil and vinegar to taste, and season as desired with sea salt and freshly ground black pepper. Serve immediately.

SALMON WITH A WATERCRESS
AND CRÈME FRAÎCHE SAUCE

Serves 4

Four 6-ounce salmon fillets
Grated zest and juice of 1 lemon
2 large sprigs fresh dill
1½ teaspoons mixed peppercorns
2 bunches fresh watercress
One 8-ounce carton (1 cup) crème fraîche
¼ cup snipped fresh chives
Sea salt and freshly ground black pepper

1. Place the salmon fillets in a single layer in a large sauté pan, and add the lemon zest and juice, dill, and peppercorns.
2. Barely cover the salmon with water, and slowly bring to a boil.
3. Remove the pan from the heat and allow the salmon to cool completely in the liquid.
4. Combine the watercress, crème fraîche, and chives in a blender or food processor and puree. Season to taste with sea salt and black pepper.
5. Lift the salmon out of the liquid, and serve with the sauce.

Poultry Main Dishes

GARDEN-FRESH STIR-FRY
WITH WATERCRESS AND CHICKEN

Serves 4

½ cup dry sherry or rice wine
2 tablespoons fresh lime juice
2 tablespoons hoisin sauce

2 teaspoons cornstarch

¼ teaspoon salt

2 tablespoons olive oil (extra-virgin is *not* recommended for stir-fry)

1 pound skinless, boneless free-range chicken breasts,
    cut into bite-size pieces

¼ cup chopped unsalted peanuts

2 teaspoons minced fresh ginger

4 carrots, thinly sliced

2 red and yellow bell peppers, thinly sliced

2 bunches B&W watercress, cut into 3-inch lengths

¼ cup chopped fresh cilantro (optional)

1. Whisk ½ cup water with the sherry, lime juice, hoisin sauce, cornstarch, and salt in a small bowl. Set the mixture aside.

2. Heat 1 tablespoon of the oil in a large skillet over medium-high heat. Add the chicken and cook, stirring occasionally, until cooked through, 4 to 6 minutes.

3. Stir in the remaining 1 tablespoon oil, the peanuts, and the ginger. Cook, stirring often, until fragrant, about 1 minute.

4. Add the carrots and bell peppers and cook, stirring constantly, for about 1 minute.

5. Whisk the sauce mixture and add it to the skillet; stir to coat. Reduce the heat to medium, cover, and cook until the vegetables are crisp-tender and the sauce has thickened, 3 to 4 minutes.

6. Stir in the watercress and cook for 1 to 2 minutes. Add the cilantro, if using, and serve.

LEMON-MINT CHICKEN CUTLETS ON WATERCRESS

Serves 3 or 4

1¼ pounds thinly sliced skinless, boneless free-range chicken breasts

1½ tablespoons grated lemon zest (from 2 lemons)

3 tablespoons fresh lemon juice

2 tablespoons olive oil

2 tablespoons chopped fresh mint, plus extra for garnish

Salt and coarsely ground black pepper

1 bag (4 ounces) B&W watercress, trimmed

1. Heat a ridged grill pan over medium-high heat (or prepare an outdoor grill for direct grilling over medium-high heat).
2. If necessary, place the chicken between sheets of plastic wrap and pound it to a uniform ¼-inch thickness.
3. In a large bowl, whisk the lemon zest, lemon juice, oil, mint, ½ teaspoon salt, and ½ teaspoon pepper until the dressing is blended. Reserve ¼ cup of the dressing.
4. Toss the chicken cutlets with the remaining dressing. Place the chicken on the grill pan (or on the outdoor grill) and cook, turning them over once, for 4 to 5 minutes.
5. To serve, toss the watercress with the reserved dressing, and divide it among 3 or 4 plates. Top with the chicken, and garnish with chopped mint.

STIR-FRY CHICKEN WITH WATERCRESS

Serves 4 to 6

¾ cup low-sodium chicken broth

2 tablespoons Chinese black bean sauce

1 tablespoon dry sherry

1 teaspoon Chinese chili-garlic sauce

2 teaspoons cornstarch

¼ cup vegetable oil

1½ pounds skinless, boneless chicken thighs, cut into ½-inch strips, or skinless, boneless breasts, cut into 1½-inch chunks

Salt and freshly ground black pepper

2 tablespoons minced fresh ginger

4 bunches B&W watercress, cut into ¾-inch pieces

1 cup fresh snow peas

1. In a small bowl, whisk the chicken broth with the black bean sauce, sherry, chili-garlic sauce, and cornstarch. Set the mixture aside.

2. Heat a large wok or skillet until very hot. Add 2 tablespoons of the vegetable oil and heat until just smoking. Season the chicken with salt and pepper, and add it to the wok in a single layer. Cook over high heat, turning once, until the chicken is browned but not cooked through, 4 to 5 minutes. Transfer the chicken to a plate and pour off the fat in the wok.

3. Add the remaining 2 tablespoons oil to the wok. Add the ginger and stir-fry until fragrant, about 30 seconds. Add the watercress and snow peas, and stir-fry until bright green and crisp-tender, 2 to 3 minutes. Return the chicken and any accumulated juices to the wok. Stir the sauce, and then add it to the wok and simmer, stirring, until thickened, about 5 minutes.

STUFFED CHICKEN BREASTS

Serves 4 to 6

3 tablespoons extra-virgin olive oil

¼ cup raisins

¼ cup pine nuts

1 tablespoon minced garlic

4 bags or bunches B&W watercress, trimmed:
    6 to 7 pretty sprigs reserved for garnish,
    the rest cut into 2- to 3-inch lengths

Salt and freshly ground black pepper

4 skinless, boneless chicken breasts (about 1½ pounds)

2 tablespoons balsamic vinegar

1 tablespoon Dijon mustard

1. Preheat the oven to 350°F. Cut six 8-inch lengths of butcher string.
2. Heat 2 tablespoons of the olive oil in a large ovenproof skillet over medium-high heat. When the oil is hot, add the raisins, pine nuts, and garlic, and cook for about 30 seconds. Then add the watercress, sprinkle with salt and pepper, and cook, stirring constantly, until the cress is wilted and fairly dry, 6 to 7 minutes. Remove and roughly chop. Set the skillet aside.
3. Place the chicken breasts on a work surface, skinned side down. Flatten them a bit with the palm of your hand, a rolling pin, or the bottom of a heavy pot. Place the watercress stuffing on top, then top with the remaining breasts, arranged so that the thick end of the top breast is over the thin end of the bottom one, so the "sandwich" is of fairly even thickness. Tie each stuffed breast in three places with the string.
4. Sprinkle the stuffed breasts on all sides with salt and pepper.
5. Heat the remaining 1 tablespoon olive oil in the same skillet you used for the stuffing, add the stuffed breasts, and sauté until browned on both sides, 5 minutes. Transfer the skillet to the oven and bake, turning the chicken once, until the chicken is cooked through and opaque, 25 to 30 minutes.
6. Transfer the chicken to a plate and tent with foil. Set the skillet over medium heat and add the vinegar, mustard, and 2 tablespoons water. Cook, stirring frequently, until the sauce is a thin syrup. Add a few grinds of black pepper.
7. Remove the string from the chicken and slice crosswise into thin or thick pieces. Serve with a spoonful of sauce drizzled over all, garnished with the reserved watercress sprigs.

PURPLE ASPARAGUS AND CHICKEN STIR-FRY*

Serves 4

15 to 20 purple or green asparagus spears, trimmed

2 tablespoons olive oil (extra-virgin is *not* recommended
   for stir-fry)

2 tablespoons minced fresh ginger

2 cloves garlic, minced

2 tablespoons finely chopped scallions, white part only

1 pound skinless, boneless chicken breasts, cubed

1 tablespoon sherry vinegar

2 teaspoons light soy sauce

25 to 30 fresh basil leaves

1 teaspoon sesame seeds

1. Cut the asparagus on the diagonal into 1-inch pieces. Set aside.
2. Heat the oil in a wok over high heat until smoking. Add the ginger,
   garlic, and scallions, and stir-fry until fragrant, about 30 seconds.
   Reduce the heat to medium-high, add the chicken, and stir-fry until
   opaque, 3 to 4 minutes. Using a wire skimmer, transfer the chicken
   to a bowl.
3. Add the asparagus to the wok and stir-fry until crisp-tender, about
   3 minutes. Add the vinegar and soy sauce, and stir to scrape up the
   browned bits. Return the chicken to the wok, add the basil, and stir-
   fry until the basil has wilted, 15 to 20 seconds.
4. Using a slotted spoon, transfer the stir-fry to a serving bowl. Sprinkle
   with the sesame seeds and serve.

Main-Dish Poultry Salads

WALDORF CHICKEN SALAD

Serves 4

3 skin-on, bone-in chicken breast halves
    (about 14 ounces each)
2 large cloves garlic, minced
1 teaspoon ground fennel seeds
Kosher salt and freshly ground black pepper
7 tablespoons extra-virgin olive oil
1 cup walnut halves
1 tablespoon red wine vinegar
½ teaspoon Dijon mustard
2 ounces blue cheese, crumbled (¼ cup)
¼ cup buttermilk
½ teaspoon finely grated lemon zest
1 cup red seedless grapes, halved
2 Fuji apples, cored and thinly sliced
2 stalks celery, thinly sliced
6 ounces B&W watercress, trimmed
2 tablespoons chopped fresh parsley
2 tablespoons chopped fresh tarragon
2 tablespoons snipped fresh chives

1. Make 3 deep slashes in each chicken breast. In a small bowl, mash
   together the garlic, fennel, 2 teaspoons salt, and pepper to taste. Stir
   in 3 tablespoons of the oil. Rub the mixture all over the chicken and
   into the slashes. Transfer the chicken to a small roasting pan, cover,
   and let stand for 1 hour.
2. Preheat the oven to 350°F.
3. Spread the walnuts in a pie plate and toast in the oven for 10 minutes,
   or until browned and fragrant. Set aside to cool.

4. Roast the chicken in the oven for about 40 minutes, or until cooked through. Let cool slightly; then discard the skin and bones, and thinly slice the meat.

5. Combine the vinegar, mustard, and remaining 4 tablespoons olive oil in a food processor, and blend. Add the blue cheese and buttermilk, and blend. Transfer to a bowl, stir in the lemon zest, and season the dressing with salt and pepper.

6. In a large bowl, combine the chicken with the walnuts, grapes, apples, celery, watercress, parsley, tarragon, and chives. Add the dressing, toss well, and serve.

WATERCRESS AND BABY ARUGULA WITH CHICKEN, GOAT CHEESE, AND PECANS

Serves 8

1 cup pecans
½ cup plus 2 tablespoons olive oil
Salt
¼ cup plus 2 tablespoons sherry vinegar
4 teaspoons Dijon mustard
½ teaspoon dried thyme
½ teaspoon dried oregano
Freshly ground black pepper
1 cooked rotisserie chicken, warm or at room temperature
9 cups loosely packed watercress, cut into 2- to 3-inch pieces
6 cups fresh baby arugula
3 cups torn fresh dandelion greens
½ red onion, sliced lengthwise into very thin strips
1 cup brined olives, such as niçoise or kalamata
⅓ cup brined capers, drained
8 ounces fresh goat cheese (may substitute feta cheese)

1. Preheat the oven to 350°F.
2. In a small bowl, combine the pecans with the 2 tablespoons olive oil and a good pinch of salt. Spread the pecans in a single layer on a baking sheet and toast for 10 to 14 minutes. Remove and set aside to cool slightly.
3. While the nuts are cooling, prepare the dressing: Pour the remaining ½ cup olive oil into a medium bowl. Whisk in the sherry vinegar, then the mustard. Whisk in the thyme, oregano, ½ teaspoon salt, and several grinds of pepper. Taste, and adjust the seasoning as desired.
4. Remove the legs and breasts from the chicken. Remove the skin, and chop the meat into coarse cubes. Set aside.
5. Combine the watercress, arugula, and dandelion greens in a large bowl. Toss in the red onion, olives, and capers, and then dress with ½ cup of the dressing. Toss the salad, adding more dressing as desired. Toss in the cubed chicken.
6. Divide the salad among 8 plates. Crumble the goat cheese in large chunks over the salads, and then sprinkle with the pecans. Serve immediately.

GREEN GRAPE, PEAR, AND DUCK SALAD

Serves 4

1 duck breast half (about 1 pound)
1 teaspoon salt
½ teaspoon freshly ground black pepper
½ teaspoon ground coriander
2 tablespoons minced shallots
2 tablespoons balsamic vinegar
2 cups seedless green grapes, some halved
2 bunches fresh watercress, stemmed (about 4 cups)
2 green pears, such as Comice or Seckel, cored and thinly sliced

1. Remove the skin and fat from the duck by pulling the fatty layer back and cutting it from the meat with a small knife. Set the breast aside.

2. Place the fatty layer, skin side down, in a skillet. Cook over medium heat, turning occasionally, until about ¼ cup of the fat has been rendered. Measure out 2 tablespoons of the fat and set it aside in the skillet. Discard the skin and the remaining fat, or save the fat for another use.

3. Raise the heat under the skillet to high. Season the duck breast on both sides with the salt, pepper, and coriander. Sear on one side until browned, about 3 minutes.

4. Turn the duck over, add the shallots, and cook for 3 minutes.

5. Reduce the heat to medium and cook the duck until it is rosy in the center, 1 to 2 minutes. Transfer it to a cutting board and tent with foil.

6. Raise the heat under the skillet to high, and add ½ cup water, the vinegar, and the whole grapes. Stir to scrape up the browned bits, and simmer until the liquid is reduced to ¼ cup, about 2 minutes.

7. Slice the duck on the diagonal into thin slices. Pour any collected juices into the skillet.

8. Arrange the watercress on a platter and top with alternating slices of pear and duck. Pour the grape sauce over, scatter the grape halves, and serve.

Beef Main Dishes

STIR-FRIED BEEF WITH BLACK BEAN SAUCE*

Serves 4

12 ounces boneless grass-fed beef sirloin
3 tablespoons olive oil (extra-virgin is *not* recommended for stir-fry)
3 tablespoons finely chopped yellow onion
2 cloves garlic, minced
6 cups packed fresh spinach leaves (1 large bunch)

2 tablespoons black bean sauce

¼ cup sherry

2 tablespoons low-sodium beef broth

Sesame seeds, for garnish

1. Cut the beef into strips 2 inches long and ¼ inch thick.
2. Heat the oil in a wok or sauté pan over high heat until almost smoking. Add the onion and stir-fry for 30 seconds. Add the garlic and stir-fry for 30 seconds. Add the beef and stir-fry until no longer red, about 3 minutes. Using a wire skimmer, transfer the ingredients to a bowl.
3. Add the spinach to the wok and stir-fry until wilted, about 1 minute. Stir in the black bean sauce, sherry, and beef broth. Return the meat mixture to the wok and stir-fry for 1 minute to heat through and coat it with the sauce. Serve hot, garnished with sesame seeds.

GRILLED STEAK SALAD
WITH GINGER-LIME DRESSING

Serves 4

¼ cup plus 2 tablespoons low-sodium soy sauce

3 tablespoons sweet chili sauce

¼ cup plus 1 tablespoon fresh lime juice

1 clove garlic, chopped

1 pound 100% grass-fed New York strip steaks

2 tablespoons rice vinegar

1 teaspoon grated fresh ginger

1 tablespoon olive oil

2 bags or bunches B&W watercress, cut into 3-inch lengths

1 cup cherry tomatoes, halved

2 carrots, chopped

1 cucumber, peeled and thinly sliced

5 radishes, sliced

1. Combine the ¼ cup soy sauce, the chili sauce, the 1 tablespoon lime juice, and the garlic in a small bowl. Place the steaks in a dish, pour the marinade over them, cover, and refrigerate for 2 hours.

2. Prepare an outdoor grill for direct grilling over medium heat (300° to 350°F).

3. In a small bowl, whisk the remaining ¼ cup lime juice with the remaining 2 tablespoons soy sauce, the vinegar, ginger, and oil. Set this dressing aside.

4. Remove the steaks from the marinade. Grill the steaks, covered with the grill lid, for 6 to 8 minutes on each side or to the desired degree of doneness. Let sit briefly before slicing. Slice across the grain into thin slices.

5. Arrange the watercress in a large bowl or on a serving platter. Top with the sliced steak, tomatoes, carrots, cucumber, and radishes. Drizzle with the ginger-lime dressing, and serve.

Brunch

WILD MUSHROOM AND GOAT CHEESE OMELETS

Serves 6 to 8 generously

6 tablespoons (¾ stick) unsalted butter

12 ounces shiitake mushrooms, stems discarded, caps thickly sliced

3 medium shallots, chopped

2 bunches fresh watercress, trimmed, cut into 3-inch lengths

Salt and freshly ground black pepper

18 large eggs

8 ounces fresh goat cheese, crumbled

1. Preheat the oven to 225°F.

2. Melt 3 tablespoons of the butter in a large skillet over medium-high heat. Add the shiitakes and cook, stirring occasionally, until golden, about 7 minutes. Add the shallots and cook until tender, about 3 minutes. Add the watercress, season with salt and pepper to taste, and cook just until the watercress is wilted, about 1 minute. Keep warm.

3. Crack 6 eggs into a medium bowl, season with salt and pepper, and beat with a whisk. Melt 1 tablespoon of the butter in a 10-inch skillet over medium-high heat. Whisk the eggs again and add them to the skillet. Cook, lifting the edges with a spatula to allow the uncooked egg to run underneath, until the bottom of the omelet is golden and the top is nearly set, about 4 minutes.

4. Spoon one-third of the mushroom filling down the center of the omelet and sprinkle with one-third of the goat cheese. Using a rubber spatula, fold the sides of the omelet over the filling to enclose it completely. Slide the omelet onto a large heatproof plate and put it in the oven to keep warm.

5. Repeat with the remaining butter, eggs, and filling to make 2 more omelets. Serve at once.

FARM EGGS
WITH WATERCRESS-PARSLEY SAUCE

Serves 5

10 large eggs, at room temperature
2 tablespoons plus ½ teaspoon kosher salt
1 small clove garlic, thinly sliced
2 tablespoons boiling water
¼ cup coarsely chopped fresh watercress
¼ cup coarsely chopped fresh flat-leaf parsley

⅛ teaspoon cayenne pepper
½ cup extra-virgin olive oil
Salt and freshly ground black pepper

1. Have ready a large bowl of ice water.
2. Place the eggs in a single layer in a large saucepan. Pour enough water over the eggs to cover by 1½ inches. Add the 2 tablespoons kosher salt and bring to a boil over high heat. Remove from the heat; cover the saucepan tightly, and let stand for 8 minutes. Drain. Return the eggs to the pan, cover with the lid, and shake the pan to crack the eggshells. Place the eggs in the ice water and cool for 5 minutes. Then peel the eggs and set them aside.
3. Place the garlic in a small ramekin. Pour the boiling water over it and let it stand for 2 minutes. Then transfer the garlic, with the liquid, to a blender. Add the watercress, parsley, cayenne, and remaining ½ teaspoon kosher salt. With the blender running, add the olive oil in a thin stream and blend until smooth. Season to taste with black pepper. (The eggs and the watercress-parsley sauce can be made 4 hours ahead. Cover separately and refrigerate. Bring the sauce to room temperature before using.)
4. Cut the eggs lengthwise into halves or quarters. If desired, cut off a very thin slice from the rounded side of each half or quarter so that the eggs can stand upright. Arrange the eggs on a platter, and sprinkle them lightly with salt and pepper. Spoon the watercress-parsley sauce over and around the eggs, and serve.

Side Dishes

SPAGHETTI SQUASH
WITH SPICED PECANS AND GORGONZOLA

This is a great side dish, and pairs nicely with a piece of grilled fish or chicken.

Serves 6 to 9

> 1 large spaghetti squash (4½ pounds),
>   halved and seeded
> 2 tablespoons plus 4 teaspoons extra-virgin olive oil
> 2 cloves garlic, minced
> 2 tablespoons coarsely chopped fresh parsley
> 2 tablespoons plus 2 teaspoons fresh lemon juice
> Salt and freshly ground black pepper
> 1 bunch fresh watercress, stems trimmed
> 2 ounces Gorgonzola cheese, crumbled (½ cup)
> Spiced Pecans (recipe follows)

1. Preheat the oven to 350°F. Line a rimmed baking sheet with a silicone baking mat or parchment paper.
2. Place the squash, cut side down, on the prepared baking sheet and bake, uncovered, for about 1 hour, until tender. Let the squash cool until it is easy to handle, and then scrape out the strands of pulp. You should have about 4 cups; set aside.
3. Heat the 2 tablespoons oil in a very large skillet over medium heat. Add the garlic and cook, stirring, for 30 seconds or until aromatic. Add the squash strands and parsley, and toss to combine. Add the 2 tablespoons lemon juice, ¼ teaspoon salt, and ¼ teaspoon pepper.
4. To serve, toss the watercress with the remaining 2 teaspoons lemon juice, remaining 4 teaspoons oil, ⅛ teaspoon salt, and ⅛ teaspoon pepper. Divide the squash mixture among individual plates or place

in a serving dish. Top with the watercress, Gorgonzola, and Spiced Pecans.

SPICED PECANS

1 egg white, lightly beaten
3 cups pecan halves
½ tablespoon salt
1 teaspoon ground cinnamon
½ teaspoon ground cloves
½ teaspoon ground nutmeg

1. Preheat the oven to 350°F. Line a baking sheet with parchment paper.
2. In a small bowl, beat the egg white with 1 tablespoon water. Stir in the pecans, mixing until well moistened.
3. Combine the salt, cinnamon, cloves, and nutmeg in a small bowl. Sprinkle the mixture over the moistened nuts. Spread the nuts on the baking sheet.
4. Bake for 30 minutes, stirring once or twice. *Be careful not to burn the nuts.* Store in the refrigerator in an airtight container until ready to use.

CHANA MASALA (SPICY CHICKPEAS) WITH WATERCRESS

Serves 4

3 tablespoons olive oil
2 cloves garlic, minced
½ onion, diced
One 16-ounce can chickpeas (also called garbanzo beans),
    or 1½ cups cooked chickpeas plus ½ cup water
Juice of 1 lemon (about 2 tablespoons)

½ teaspoon curry powder
½ teaspoon ground coriander
½ teaspoon ground cumin
½ teaspoon garam masala
1 large bunch or 2 handfuls fresh watercress, trimmed

1. Heat the oil in a large skillet or sauté pan over medium heat. Add the onion and garlic, and sauté until soft, 3 to 5 minutes. Add the chickpeas straight from the can, including all the liquid. Add the lemon juice and spices, cover, and simmer, stirring occasionally, adding more water if needed, until the chickpeas are browned and soft, 10 to 15 minutes.

2. Reduce the heat, add the watercress, and cover. Cook until the watercress has wilted, 2 to 4 minutes. Serve immediately.

BRAISED MIXED GREENS

Escarole, trimmed and coarsely chopped
Kale, trimmed and coarsely chopped
Swiss chard, trimmed and coarsely chopped
Spinach, trimmed and coarsely chopped
Extra-virgin olive oil
Minced garlic
Salt and freshly ground black pepper

1. Toss the escarole, kale, chard, and spinach together in a large bowl.

2. Combine the greens and water in a large sauté pan and cook, stirring, until they are limp, 3 to 5 minutes. Drain well.

3. Wipe the pan dry and place it over medium heat. Add the olive oil, drained greens, garlic, and salt and pepper to taste. Cover, and cook briefly until soft.

SAVORY BROCCOLI SAUTÉ*

Olive oil
Small broccoli florets
Chopped pitted green olives
Brined capers, drained
Grated lemon zest
Crushed red pepper flakes
Cloves garlic, thinly sliced

1. Heat the oil in a sauté pan over medium heat. Add the broccoli and cook, letting the florets sizzle, until softened.
2. Add the olives, capers, lemon zest, red pepper flakes, and garlic, and sauté until the broccoli is golden and the flavors have melded.

ROAST BRUSSELS SPROUTS*

Brussels sprouts
Olive oil
Salt and freshly ground black pepper
Minced fresh oregano or thyme

1. Preheat the oven to 350°F.
2. Peel away the outer leaves of the brussels sprouts, and trim the stems. Cut the sprouts in half.
3. In a mixing bowl, combine the brussels sprouts, oil, salt and pepper to taste, and the oregano. Toss to coat.
4. Place the mixture in a baking dish and roast in the oven, turning occasionally, until the sprouts are golden and fork-tender, 40 minutes.

WATERCRESS AMANDINE

Serves 4

1 tablespoon unsalted butter
¼ cup slivered almonds
8 bunches fresh watercress, trimmed
Sea salt and freshly ground black pepper

1. Melt the butter in a heavy nonstick skillet over medium-high heat. Add the almonds and sauté for 3 to 4 minutes, until golden. Transfer the almonds to a bowl.
2. Add the watercress to the skillet, cover tightly, and cook, stirring occasionally, until it wilts, 2 to 3 minutes.
3. Stir in the buttered almonds. Season with sea salt and black pepper to taste, and serve.

WILTED WATERCRESS WITH ROASTED GARLIC

Serves 6

12 cloves garlic, peeled
4 tablespoons olive oil
4 bunches or bags B&W watercress, cut into 3-inch pieces
Salt and freshly ground black pepper

1. Preheat the oven to 400°F.
2. Place the garlic cloves on a piece of foil, and drizzle with 1 tablespoon of the oil. Wrap the garlic up in the foil and roast until soft, about 20 minutes.
3. Heat the remaining 3 tablespoons oil in a large pot over medium-high heat. Add the watercress and the garlic, with the oil, from the foil packet. Sauté until the watercress has wilted, about 2 minutes. Season with salt and pepper to taste. Transfer the watercress to a bowl, and serve.

KASHA*

1 cup kasha
1 large egg, well beaten
1 tablespoon olive oil
Sea salt, to taste
Chopped fresh parsley, for garnish

1. Stir the kasha and egg together in a small bowl.
2. Heat the olive oil in a sauté pan over medium-high heat. Add the kasha mixture and cook, stirring to separate the grains, until toasted, 3 to 5 minutes.
3. Add 2 cups water and a little sea salt, cover, and cook over medium heat until fluffy, about 15 minutes. Serve, garnished with chopped parsley.

SHIITAKES SAUTÉED WITH GARLIC*

Shiitake mushrooms, stemmed
Minced garlic
Sea salt and freshly ground black pepper
Minced fresh parsley
Olive oil

1. Quarter the shiitake mushroom caps and place them in a bowl. Sprinkle with the garlic, sea salt and black pepper to taste, and parsley, and toss to mix.
2. Heat the olive oil in a sauté pan over low heat, add the mushrooms, and sauté until they are just beginning to crisp, 10 to 15 minutes. Serve immediately.

CAULIFLOWER GRATIN*

Serves 4

Butter, for the baking dish
1 head cauliflower, cored and cut into large florets
1 tablespoon olive oil
2 ounces pancetta, chopped
1 yellow onion, thinly sliced
½ teaspoon freshly ground black pepper
4 ounces Muenster cheese, thinly sliced

1. Preheat the oven to 350°F. Butter a baking dish that is just large enough to hold the cauliflower in a single layer.
2. Bring water to a simmer in the bottom of a vegetable steamer. Place the cauliflower in the steamer basket, cover, and steam until fork-tender, 10 to 15 minutes. Transfer the cauliflower to the prepared baking dish.
3. Heat the oil in a sauté pan over medium heat. Add the pancetta and onion, and sauté until the pancetta is crisp and the onion is golden, about 15 minutes.
4. Spoon the pancetta mixture over the cauliflower and sprinkle with the pepper. Top with the cheese slices, covering the surface evenly. Bake until the edges are bubbling, about 20 minutes. Serve hot.

Salads

WARM MIXED BEAN SALAD
WITH PANCETTA ON WATERCRESS

This delectable warm bean salad is based on the inspired creation of a chef at one of my favorite Italian restaurants, Centro, in Fairfield, Connecticut.

Roman beans are large, relatively soft-textured beans used extensively in Italian cooking. They are pretty widely available in New England as well as around the rest of the country, but if you can't find them, the ubiquitous kidney bean will do just fine.

Pancetta is Italian bacon that has been cured with salt and spices, but is not smoked. It is available in Italian markets and many supermarkets.

Serves 4

6 tablespoons plus 2 teaspoons extra-virgin olive oil
⅓ cup (1½ ounces) diced pancetta or
    diced thick-sliced preservative-free bacon
4 cloves garlic, peeled and crushed until flat (see Note)
One 10-ounce package frozen lima beans,
    cooked and drained
1½ cups drained canned Roman or red kidney beans
1½ cups drained canned black beans
2 tablespoons fresh lemon juice
2 bags or bunches B&W watercress, trimmed
¼ teaspoon freshly ground black pepper
Salt
3 tablespoons chopped fresh flat-leaf parsley,
    plus sprigs for garnish
1 lemon, cut into 4 wedges

1. Warm the 2 teaspoons olive oil in a large skillet over low heat. Add the pancetta and cook until crisp and any fat is rendered, about 10 minutes. Remove the pancetta with a slotted spoon and reserve. Pour the fat out of the skillet but do not wash the skillet.
2. Add the remaining 6 tablespoons oil and the garlic to the skillet. Cook over low heat until the garlic turns a pale golden brown, watching carefully so it doesn't scorch, about 10 minutes. Remove the garlic with tongs, leaving the oil in the skillet.

3. Add the lima beans, Roman beans, and black beans to the garlic oil in the skillet, raise the heat to medium-high, and toss gently until heated through, about 4 minutes. Add the pancetta and lemon juice, and stir gently to combine. Add 1 bag of the watercress and cook until wilted, 1 to 2 minutes. Season with the black pepper and salt to taste. (The salad may not need salt, as the pancetta or bacon is salty.)

4. Spread the remaining 1 bag watercress out on a serving platter or on individual plates. Spoon the warm beans over the watercress and sprinkle with the parsley. Garnish with the lemon wedges and parsley sprigs, and serve.

NOTE: This salad is flavored rather subtly with garlic. For a more assertive garlic flavor, mince 1 or 2 of the cooked cloves and stir them into the finished salad.

WHITE BEAN AND ASPARAGUS SALAD WITH WATERCRESS

Serves 4

5 stalks green asparagus, tough ends removed
One 15-ounce can white beans (such as cannellini),
    rinsed and drained
1 orange bell pepper, seeded and chopped
½ cup finely chopped red onion
2 tablespoons extra-virgin olive oil
2 tablespoons fresh lemon juice
1 teaspoon Dijon mustard
Salt and freshly ground black pepper
2 cups B&W watercress, trimmed

1. Bring water to a simmer in a vegetable steamer.
2. Cut the asparagus into 1-inch pieces, place them in the steamer basket, cover, and lightly steam, 2 to 3 minutes. Set aside to cool.

3. In a large bowl, combine the white beans, bell pepper, and red onion. Add the asparagus and toss gently. In a separate bowl, whisk together the olive oil, lemon juice, mustard, and salt and pepper to taste. Gently toss the dressing into the salad and adjust the seasoning.

4. Line a salad bowl with the watercress, and top with the white bean salad.

KIDNEY BEAN AND TARRAGON SALAD*

Champagne vinegar
Dijon mustard
Extra-virgin olive oil
15-ounce cans red kidney beans, drained and rinsed
Minced fresh tarragon
Chopped red onion
Sea salt and freshly ground black pepper

Combine the vinegar and mustard in a large bowl. Whisk in the olive oil until emulsified. Add the beans, tarragon, and onion. Season with sea salt and pepper to taste, and mix to combine.

CELERY ROOT, RADISH, AND WATERCRESS SALAD WITH MUSTARD SEED DRESSING

Thanks to the mustard seeds, mustard, watercress, and radishes, your mitochondrial DNA will love this cruciferous veggie delight!

Serves 8

1 tablespoon yellow mustard seeds
½ cup white balsamic vinegar
1 tablespoon Dijon mustard
¼ cup minced shallots (2 medium shallots)

⅔ cup extra-virgin olive oil

Sea salt and freshly ground black pepper

2 large bunches fresh watercress, thick stems trimmed
(about 6 cups packed)

1½ pounds celery root (also called celeriac),
trimmed, peeled, and coarsely grated in a food processor
or with a box grater

20 radishes, trimmed and thinly sliced

1. Place a dry skillet over medium heat, add the mustard seeds, and stir until they are lightly toasted and starting to pop, about 3 minutes. Transfer the mustard seeds to a bowl and let them cool.
2. Add the vinegar, mustard, and shallots to the cooled mustard seeds; whisk to blend. Gradually whisk in the oil. Season with sea salt and black pepper to taste.
3. In a large bowl, toss the watercress with enough of the dressing to coat it lightly. Divide the watercress among 8 plates.
4. Combine the celery root and radishes in the same bowl; toss with enough of the remaining dressing to coat. Season with sea salt and pepper to taste. Top the watercress with the celery root mixture, and serve.

CRISP ESCAROLE-WATERCRESS SALAD
WITH GARLICKY ANCHOVY DRESSING

Anchovies are the chefs' (and health and beauty seekers') best-kept secret. They add the most delicious flavor to a huge number of dishes, including the world-famous Caesar salad. And they are high in the skin-firming nutrient DMAE.

Serves 4

1 large head escarole, light green and white leaves only,
cut crosswise into 1-inch-wide strips

1 bunch or bag B&W watercress, cut into 2- to 3-inch lengths

6 radishes, trimmed and thinly sliced

4 stalks celery with leaves, thinly sliced

1 cup grape tomatoes, halved

½ seedless cucumber, halved lengthwise and
thinly sliced crosswise

½ cup extra-virgin olive oil

8 oil-packed anchovy fillets, drained and coarsely chopped

6 large cloves garlic, minced

2½ tablespoons fresh lemon juice

Freshly ground black pepper

Sea salt

1. In a large bowl, toss the escarole and watercress with the radishes, celery, tomatoes, and cucumber.
2. Combine the olive oil, chopped anchovies, and minced garlic in a small saucepan over moderate heat, and cook, stirring occasionally, until the garlic is lightly golden, about 7 minutes. Add the lemon juice and season generously with pepper.
3. Pour the warm dressing over the salad, season lightly with sea salt, and toss again. Serve at once.

A Final Word

If you follow the guidelines outlined in the preceding chapters, you will see that the program set forth in these pages is not difficult to follow, nor is it expensive, requiring costly and sometimes dangerous prescription drugs. Although the results are cumulative and continue to accrue the longer you follow the program, you will notice changes in your body and mind within a few days. These positive changes include an elevation of mood, a newfound optimism, loss of body fat, increased skin radiance, and unbounded energy to accomplish your daily tasks. Too much body fat, wrinkled and sagging skin, and an addled mental state can all be transformed.

The goal of this book is to provide you with all the tools and guidance you need to ensure success, regardless of your age. You can do this by applying the dietary and nutritional strategies presented in these pages to minimize the triple threat of inflammation, glycation, and oxidative stress. The results you can look forward to include a revitalized face and body, increased stamina and energy, improved memory and brainpower, decreased body fat, and increased muscle mass.

The anti-inflammatory diet, targeted nutritional substances, a new generation of topical treatments, and the power of yoga to rejuvenate mind and body will work together synergistically to keep you Forever Young—or at least looking and feeling significantly younger than your chronological age.

Acknowledgments

Anne Sellaro again deserves star billing in these acknowledgments. Anne's untiring enthusiasm, hard work, loyalty, creativity, and vision as friend, agent, producer, and collaborator continue to help me share my message and mission with millions of people worldwide.

I would like to extend a warm thank-you to the great many friends and colleagues who have generously assisted me, including the outstanding team at Atria, a division of Simon & Schuster. It has been a great joy and privilege working with this team of professionals, starting with our exceptional editor, Emily Bestler, and the wonderful editorial, publicity, marketing, and sales experts:

Emily Bestler, VP and Executive Editorial Director
Laura Stern, Assistant Editor
Kate Cetrulo, Editorial Assistant
Judith Curr, Publisher
Chris Lloreda, Associate Publisher
Rachel Sciambra, Publicity Manager
Jeanne Lee, Art Director
Michael Selleck, Executive VP, Sales and Marketing
Lisa Keim, Subsidiary Rights Director
Paula Amendolara, Senior Director, National Accounts
Colin Shields, Director, National Sales
Janice Fryer, National Accounts Manager
Lauren Monaco, VP Sales, National Accounts
Gary Urda, VP Sales

Jessica Ko, National Accounts Manager
Liz Perl, SVP, Director of Marketing
Susan Reed, Publicity Director

Other colleagues and friends indispensable to the success of this project
include:

Diane Miles, CEO and President, Perricone MD
Daniel Giles, Senior VP, Marketing and Creative, Perricone MD
David Vigliano and the team at Vigliano Associates
Diane Reverand
Diti Katona and John Pylypczak,
    Concrete Design and Communication
Wini Linguvic
Tony Tiano, Lennlee Keep, Jim Hoppin, Eli Brown,
    and the team at Santa Fe Productions
The Public Broadcasting Service (PBS-TV)
Harry G. Preuss, M.D., M.A.C.N., C.N.S.
Stephen Sinatra, M.D., F.A.C.N., F.A.C.C.
Michigan State University College of Human Medicine
Department of Dermatology, Henry Ford Hospital
Mitsunori Nishida, President and CEO of Fuji Chemical,
    Charles DePrince (President and CEO) and Yasuko Kuroda
    of Fuji Health Sciences, Inc., our astaxanthin experts
Bob Terry, Ph.D., Technical Service Adviser, and Jason Nava,
    EVP, Green Foods Corporation
Richard and Pat Burgoon, Andy Brown of
    B&W Quality Growers
Mike Shirota, Shuji Matsubara, and Donna Noonan of
    Mushroom Wisdom
Frank Assumma and Cheryl Costanzo of Natural Health
    Science Inc. and Frank Schonlau, Ph.D., Horphag
    Research Ltd (UK), our Pycnogenol® experts

Kella England and the team at the NV Perricone MD
    Flagship Store
The team at Perricone MD
Edward Magnotti
Terence Sellaro
Johnna Schlosser
Chim Potini
Parker Ladd
Vincent Perricone
Jon Morrow
Jeff Hurley
Maria La Rosa
Ed and Eve Hoffmann
St. Regis Hotel management and staff
Lou Anna K. Simon, President, Michigan State University
Steve Kaplan, President, University of New Haven
Craig Weatherby, Randy and Carla Hartnell,
    and the team at Vital Choice
Steve Oates
Williams-Sonoma
My mother
My children, Jeffrey, Nicholas, and Caitie
My brother and sisters, Jimmy, Laura, Barbara, and June

Resources

To receive updates on the latest health, beauty, and antiaging news (and more) visit www.perriconemd.com.

To receive updates on the latest health, beauty, and antiaging news featured in Forever Young, visit www.perriconemd.com and sign up to receive our newsletter.

Perricone MD skin care system— a skin care system customized to your individual needs.

Rx1: Prevent Kit
Rx2: Correct Kit
Rx3: Repair Kit
Rx4: Restore Kit

Perricone MD Hand Held Microcurrent

Targeted Care

Skin Clear (Skin Clear Cleanser, Skin Clear Toner, Skin Clear Hydrator, and Skin Clear Supplements)

- º www.perriconemd.com or contact our skin care specialist at 1-888-823-7837
- º N. V. Perricone, M.D., flagship store at 791 Madison Avenue (at East 67th Street), New York, NY 10021
- º Sephora, www.sephora.com
- º QVC, www.qvc.com
- º Nordstrom, www.nordstrom.com
- º Neiman Marcus, www.neimanmarcus.com

Perricone MD Nutriceuticals

Vitamin C Ester

Alpha Lipoic Acid

DMAE

Maitake Mushroom Extract

Omega-3

PEP

Chia seeds

Watercress

Perricone Super Antioxidant

Pigment Corrective

Health & Weight Management

Skin & Total Body

Superberry Powder with Acai

o   www.perriconemd.com or contact our skin care specialist at
1-888-823-7837

o   N. V. Perricone, M.D., flagship store at 791 Madison Avenue
(at East 67th Street), New York, NY 10021

o   Sephora, www.sephora.com

o   QVC, www.qvc.com

o   Nordstrom, www.nordstrom.com

o   Neiman Marcus, www.neimanmarcus.com

AstaREAL Astaxanthin Supplements

CAN-C Carnosine Eye Drops

IAS (International Aging Systems) Group, www.antiaging-medicine.com.

Pyridoxamine, the rare antiaging B vitamin

IAS Group, www.antiaging-medicine.com.

Rhodiola—Arctic Root

Arctic Root is made from a unique extract of *Rhodiola rosea* (SHR-5)
and developed for stress relief, mental clarity, energy, and positive mood

support. There is only one Arctic Root, produced after thirty years of research, clinical trials, and safety studies by the Swedish Herbal Institute. For more information and to order, visit www.proactivebio .com.

Supplements for Bone Health and Cardiovascular Support

Vitamin K2

- Vitamin K2/bone solutions, Advanced Biosolutions, 888-887-7498 or www.drsinatra.com.
- Choline-stabilized orthosilicic acid (ch-OSA), Jarrow Formulas BioSil, www.jarrow.com.

P 73 Oreganol and Related Products

Oil of oregano is an herbal product that has been used since biblical times. It was widely used in ancient Greece for many medical purposes. Oil of oregano is a potent antiseptic, meaning it kills germs. Research proves that it is highly effective for killing a wide range of fungi, yeast, and bacteria, including MRSA and avian bird flu, as well as parasites and viruses.

- North American Herb & Spice, 800-243-5242 or www.oreganol.com.

Starch and Sugar Blockers

Wild Alaskan salmon/tuna/halibut/sardines; wild organic blueberries; organic dark chocolate; organic herbs and spices; organic teas; salmon sausage and burgers.

- Vital Choice Wild Alaskan salmon has a healthier fatty acid profile (less saturated fat, higher ratio of omega-3 fatty acids to saturated fats), than farmed salmon. Vital Choice Seafood products (salmon, tuna, and halibut) are caught at sea, flash-frozen immediately, packed in dry ice, and delivered by FedEx or UPS at affordable prices. In 2000, it was the first fishery certified sustainable by the Marine Stewardship Council. 800-608-4825 or www.vitalchoice.com.

Açai (Amazonian fruit high in antioxidants)

○ Açai fruit has more antioxidants than wild blueberries, pomegranates, or red wine; it also contains essential omegas (healthy fats), amino acids, calcium, and fiber.

Super Berry Powder with Açai

A berry powder drink containing high amounts of antioxidants and anti-inflammatories. Both qualities maintain cell health and protection from free-radical damage, and provide support to the major organ functions in the body. Contains açai, ranked as the number one superfood in Dr. Perricone's book *The Perricone Promise.*

○ N. V. Perricone, M.D., 888-823-7837, www.perriconemd.com

○ N. V. Perricone, M.D., flagship store, 791 Madison Avenue (at East 67th Street) New York, 10021

○ Sambazon brand açai beverages can also be found nationwide at Whole Foods Market and Wild Oats stores, www.sambazon.com.

Avocados

Recipes and health information: The California Avocado Commission, www.avocado.org.

Beans and Lentils

Westbrae Naturals markets certified-organic beans, including rare "heirloom" varieties, nationwide, 800-434-4246, www.westbrae.com/products/index.html.

Coconut Oil

Garden of Life Extra Virgin Coconut Oil
866-465-0051
www.gardenoflife.com

Foods Alive Organic Golden Flax Crackers (Grain-Free)

Foods Alive, www.foodsalive.com

Organic Dairy Products and Cheeses

Organic Valley is organic and farmer-owned since 1988. This co-op of more than 1,100 farmers produces the finest organic products, including milk, yogurt, and cheeses. Widely available in natural food stores and the natural food section of your supermarket, www.organicvalley .coop.

Goat and Sheep Dairy Products

Redwood Hill Farms

This company's delicious goat milk yogurt and fine artisanal cheeses are a natural in cooking. Try using Redwood Hill Farm Goat Milk Yogurt in almost any recipe that calls for milk, cream, sour cream, or buttermilk. Redwood Hill Farm cheeses, fresh or aged, soft or crumbly, spreadable or hard, are perfect for any course. Goat cheese, like goat milk, is easier on the human digestive system and lower in calories, cholesterol, and fat than its bovine counterpart. Goat cheese is rich in calcium, protein, vitamin A, vitamin K, phosphorus, niacin, and thiamine. The company's Web site, www.redwoodhill.com, also has great recipes.

The Coonridge Organic Goat Cheese Dairy

Since 1981, Coonridge Organic Goat Cheese has been altering the dynamics of natural cheeses. It offers a selection with superior flavor and full nutrition in reusable packaging. Coonridge proves that wonderful taste and nutritional superiority doesn't have to come at the expense of the environment, the goat's health, or our health. Besides promoting sustainable, nonchemical, non-factory-farmed animal husbandry and cheese making, they strive to always live in harmony with the natural world that supports us all. www.coonridge.com.

Feta Cheese

Malincho has outstanding goat feta from the Balkans that is tremendously flavorful—and many other products as well. Order at 866-203-3525 or www.malincho.com.

**Grating Cheeses from Italy,
Including Pecorino Romano and Parmigiano-Reggiano**
From the high mountains of Valle d'Aosta through the foggy Piedmont, on to Tuscany and the islands of Sicily and Sardinia, Italy's cheeses offer variety not only in size and shape but in texture and flavor as well. http://formaggio-kitchen.com.

Premium artisan cheeses from around the world: www.gourmet library.com

Raw Milk Aged Cheddar Cheese

My personal favorite is **Shelburne Farms** Three Year Cheddar. On the beautiful shores of Lake Champlain in Burlington, Vermont, all the milking cows in their purebred herd of Brown Swiss are raised on the farm and graze on pasture from spring to fall. Shelburne Farms own milk—absolutely fresh, untreated, and rbST/rbGH free—is used to make their award-winning cheese. The only other cheese ingredients are starter culture, rennet, and salt. www.shelburnefarms.org.

Kefir and Yogurt

Helios Nutrition is a small organic dairy in Sauk Centre, Minnesota, that makes several flavors of organic kefir with added FOS (a prebiotic polysaccharide). 888-3-HELIOS (343-5467) or www.heliosnutrition .com.

Stonyfield Farm yogurt is available at many food markets, www.stony field.com/Store.finder/index.jsp.

Horizon Organic yogurt is available at many food markets, www .horizondairy.com/static/pop_locator.html.

Diamond Organics sells organic yogurt direct to consumers at www .diamondorganics.com.

For excellent information on many topics, including raw milk cheeses, visit the Weston A. Price Foundation at www.realmilk.com.

100% Grass-Fed Beef

For superb all-natural beef from the pristine countryside of Vermont:

Vermont Natural Beef
1943 Stage Road
Benson, VT 05743
802-537-3711
www.vermontnaturalbeef.com

Eatwild.com is your source for safe, healthy, natural, and nutritious grass-fed beef, lamb, goat, bison, poultry, pork, and dairy products. The site has three goals:

○ To link consumers with reliable suppliers of all-natural, delicious, grass-fed products

○ To provide comprehensive, accurate information about the benefits of raising animals on pasture

○ To provide a marketplace for farmers who raise their livestock on pasture from birth to market and who actively promote the welfare of their animals and the health of the land

www.eatwild.com

Green Foods

Certified organic barley grass, Green Magma powder, and supplements. Available at natural food stores including Whole Foods and Wild Oats. For additional retailers and online retailers, visit www.greenfoods.com.

Green Tea

Red Blossom Tea Co.
831 Grant Avenue
San Francisco, CA 94108-1708
415-395-0868
www.redblossomtea.com

Green Tea Extract

The active constituents in green tea are polyphenols, with an antioxidant called epigallocatechin-3-gallate (EGCG) being the most powerful. You can find many products in drug and natural food stores listed as either green tea extract or EGCG. Life Extension has a Mega Green Tea Extract available at www.lef.org.

Organic Fruits and Vegetables Delivered to Your Home

Diamond Organics sells certified-organic berries (in season, May through October) direct to consumers, 888-ORGANIC (888-674-2642) or www.diamondorganics.com.

Organic Markets Nationwide

For fish, meat, poultry, eggs, fruits and vegetables, barley, oats, buckwheat, beans and lentils, hot peppers, nuts, seeds, extra-virgin olive oil, herbs, spices, spring water, tea (green, white, and black), nutritional supplements, kefir, yogurt, and other products.

Whole Foods Market has an outstanding choice of natural and organic foods, www.wholefoods.com.

Polysaccharide Peptide Food Products
(anti-inflammatory and antiaging)

- N. V. Perricone, M.D., 888-823-7837 or www.perriconemd.com
- N. V. Perricone, M.D., Flagship Store at 791 Madison Avenue (at East 67th Street), New York, NY 10021

Pistachio Nuts

California pistachio nuts, www.everybodysnuts.com. Found in supermarkets and grocery stores nationwide.

Pomegranate Juice and Concentrate (extremely high in antioxidants)

POM Wonderful, 310-966-5800 or www.pomwonderful.com. Also available at supermarkets and natural food stores.

Pure Spring Water

o **Poland Spring,** found in supermarkets and grocery stores nationwide.

o **FIJI Water** natural artesian water bottled at its source in the Fijian islands. Available at leading grocery and convenience chains. FIJI Water is also available for home delivery in the continental United States, www.fijiwater.com.

Sea Vegetables

o **Maine Coast Sea Vegetables,** www.seaveg.com

o **Eden Foods,** www.edenfoods.com

Sprouts: Information and Supplies

o The International Sprout Growers Association (ISGA) is the professional association of sprout growers and companies, which supplies products and services to the sprout industry. Visit www.isga-sprouts.org for outstanding information, recipes, and health notes.

o Another first-class site for information and products is www.sproutpeople.net.

Turmeric Extract

o **New Chapter** markets the high-potency turmeric extract TurmericForce, 800-543-7279 or www.new-chapter.com.

o Most natural food stores and grocers also carry fresh turmeric root.

Recommended Cookware and Bakeware

It should come as no surprise that my favorite cookware and bakeware hails from France, one of the countries most famed for superior cuisine. The cookware that you choose is very important to your health as well as to the flavor of your food. Porcelain and enameled cookware will not interact with your food, which is important to know when you are dealing with acidic foods such as vinegar and lemon. As mentioned, avoid nonstick cookware and bakeware. Although the recommended items cost a bit more, properly cared for they will last a lifetime—a wise investment that you have to make only once.

Emile Henry Cookware

Since 1850 five generations of the Henry family have been handcrafting this famous oven-to-tableware in the Burgundy region in the heart of France. Emile Henry is the largest manufacturer of pottery in France. Since it was first produced, the major benefit of cooking in oven-to-tableware has been its ability to allow gradual, even heat distribution throughout the food so the fibers soften slowly, without toughening. Available at fine stores such as Williams-Sonoma. For complete retail and online listings, visit www.emilehenry.com.

Le Creuset

Le Creuset is the world's leading manufacturer of enameled cast-iron cookware. Like Emile Henry, Le Creuset is as beautiful as it is functional. The only challenge when it comes to shopping for Le Creuset is choosing the color. All Le Creuset cookware is made from enameled cast iron. Cast iron has been used for cooking utensils since the Middle Ages. The Le Creuset factory is at Fresnoy-le-Grand in northern France. In 1925, the foundry began hand-casting molten cast iron in sand molds, still the most delicate stage of the production process. Even today, after casting, each mold is destroyed and the cookware is polished and sanded by hand, then scrutinized for imperfections. Once declared good for enameling, the items are sprayed with two separate coats of enamel and fired after each process at a temperature of 800°C. The enamel then becomes extremely hard and durable, making it almost completely resistant to damage during normal use. Since much of the finishing is done by hand, each Le Creuset cast-iron cookware piece is completely unique. Visit www.lecreuset.com.

Recommended Household Products

Seventh Generation

There is an alternative to toxic cleansers and environmentally unfriendly paper and plastic. I recommend Seventh Generation, which offers a complete line of nontoxic household products. All of its products are designed to work as well as their traditional counterparts but use renewable, nontoxic, phosphate free, and biodegradable ingredients and are never tested on animals. They are as gentle on the planet as they are on people, and they don't create fumes or leave residues that may affect the health of your family or your pets. Seventh Generation products are widely available nationwide. To learn more and find a retailer or online retailer, visit www.seventhgeneration.com.

Health Education Information

These Web sites offer interesting information on the topics of nutrition, natural healing, food, and holistic health.

IAS Group

An outstanding source for antiaging medicine, nutrition, and information, www.antiaging-systems.com.

Life Extension

For up-to-the-minute scientific news and information on food and nutritional supplements, including the latest on the weight loss benefits of sesame seeds, www.lef.org.

European Food Information Council (EUFIC)

EUFIC is a nonprofit organization that provides science-based information on food and food-related topics to the media, health and nutrition professionals, educators, and opinion leaders, www.eufic.org.

The Glycemic Index

For information on the glycemic index, www.glycemicindex.com.

Mercola.com

For excellent information on general health and nutrition, including different types of meat, sugars, and so on, www.mercola.com.

The American Institute for Cancer Research

For information on the cancer-preventing phytonutrients found in fruits and vegetables, www.aicr.org.

President's Council on Physical Fitness and Sports (PCPFS)
The National Institute on Aging

For outstanding information on the benefits and various types of exercise, including detailed information with drawings, visit the following Web sites: www.fitness.gov, www.niapublications.org.

Health Benefits of Olive Oil

International Olive Oil Council, www.internationaloliveoil.com

Nonglycemic Sweeteners

To learn more about the pros and cons of all of the available sweeteners, both natural and chemical, visit www.holisticmed.com/sweet, Stevia .net, www.stevia.net.

Soy Foods

U.S. Soyfoods Directory, www.soyfoods.com

Seafood Safety

Environmental Protection Agency (EPA)
www.epa.gov/ost/fish, www.epa.gov/mercury

Union of Concerned Scientists
www.ucsusa.org

U.S. Food and Drug Administration
Food safety Web site, www.cfsan.fda.gov/~frf/sea-mehg.html

Yoga and Fitness

Wini Linguvic
www.bodychange.com
info@bodychange.com

For outstanding results-oriented fitness, I highly recommend Wini Linguvic's programs:

BodyChange Kick-Start

BodyChange Balance

Strength and Conditioning for Yogis

Recommended Reading

Ageless Face, Ageless Mind: Erase Wrinkles & Rejuvenate the Brain, Nicholas Perricone, M.D., Ballantine Books, New York, 2007.

Dr. Perricone's 7 Secrets to Beauty, Health, and Longevity, Nicholas Perricone, M.D., Ballantine Books, New York, 2006.

The Perricone Weight-Loss Diet, Nicholas Perricone, M.D., Ballantine Books, New York, 2005.

The Perricone Promise, Nicholas Perricone, M.D., Warner Books, New York, 2004.

The Clear Skin Prescription, Nicholas Perricone, M.D., HarperCollins, New York, 2003.

The Perricone Prescription, Nicholas Perricone, M.D., HarperCollins, New York, 2002.

The Wrinkle Cure, Nicholas Perricone, M.D., Warner Books, New York, 2001.

Barley Grass Juice: Rejuvenation Elixir and Natural, Healthy Power Drink, Barbara Simonsohn, Lotus Press, Twin Lakes, Wis., 2001.

Green Barley Essence: The Ideal Fast Food, Dr. Yoshihide Hagiwara, McGraw-Hill, Hightstown, N.J., 1985.

Green Leaves of Barley: Nature's Miracle Rejuvenator, Dr. Mary Ruth Swope and David A. Darbro, M.D., Swope Enterprises, Lone Star, Texas, 1996.

Maitake Magic, Harry Preuss, M.D., M.A.C.N., C.N.S., and Sensuke Konno, Freedom Publishing Company, Evanston, Ill., 2002.

Natural Cures for Killer Germs and *The Cure Is in the Cupboard*, Dr. Cass Ingram, Knowledge House Publishers, Vernon Hills, Ill., revised edition, 2008.

The Natural Weight Loss Pharmacy, Harry Preuss, M.D., M.A.C.N., C.N.S., and Bill Gottlieb, Broadway Books, New York, 2007.

The Omnivore's Dilemma, Michael Pollan, Penguin Press, New York, 2006.

Pasture Perfect: The Far-Reaching Benefits of Choosing Meat, Eggs, and Dairy Products from Grass-Fed Animals, Jo Robinson, available at www.eatwild.com.

Wheat Grass: Nature's Finest Medicine, Steve Meyerowitz, Sproutman Publications, Great Barrington, Mass., 1998.

   This book is actually about cereal grasses, not just wheat grass, and it contains a large section of scientific research on the health benefits of barley grass juice.

Index